BROKE

Patients Talk about Money with Their Doctor

MICHAEL STEIN, M.D.

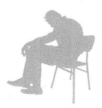

The University of North Carolina Press

CHAPEL HILL

This book was published with the assistance of the Lilian R. Furst Fund of the University of North Carolina Press.

© 2020 Michael Stein
Manufactured in the United States of America

Designed and set by Kim Bryant in Whitman and Real Head Pro types

The University of North Carolina Press has been a member of the Green Press Initiative since 2003.

Cover illustration: © Shutterstock.com/ Vladimir Sviracevic.

Library of Congress Cataloging-in-Publication Data

Names: Stein, Michael, 1960– author.

Title: Broke: patients talk about money with their doctor / Michael Stein, M.D.

Description: Chapel Hill: The University of North Carolina Press, 2020.

Identifiers: LCCN 2020016435 | ISBN 9781469661131 (cloth : alk. paper) |

ISBN 9781469661148 (pbk. : alk. paper) |

ISBN 9781469661155 (ebook)

Subjects: LCSH: Medical economics—United States. | Poor—Health and hygiene—United States. | Poor—Medical care—United States.

Classification: LCC RA410.53 .S744 2020 |

DDC 338.4/73621—dc23

LC record available at https://lccn.loc.gov/2020016435

BROKE

ALSO BY MICHAEL STEIN

FICTION

Probabilities

The White Life

The Lynching Tree

In the Age of Love

This Room Is Yours

The Rape of the Muse

NONFICTION

The Lonely Patient

The Addict: One Patient, One Doctor, One Year

Pained: Uncomfortable Conversations about the Public's Health

To Peter Kramer, friend, walker, reader, writer

Contents

A Note to the Reader

This book contains the stories of real people who have agreed to share their thoughts and struggles with me. My patients share their stories in confidence, and I must honor that trust. I have changed names and genders and family members, changed places, and conveyed few physical descriptions of the speakers. In many cases I have created composites to protect anonymity. I hope to disguise; anyone recognizable is coincidental.

BROKE

Introduction

I get asked for lots of things in my office: pain medications, referrals, refills, a few more minutes. My medical office is in a poor neighborhood. In twenty-five years, I have never been asked for money by a patient.

Recently, with the country seemingly getting richer, my patients find themselves getting poorer, and with a president dividing the world into the deserving and undeserving, I'm finding that I spend a lot of time talking about money with the people who come to see me—though lack of money is never their presenting complaint. And it doesn't happen right away—they arrive with the medical problems an internist is trained to hear and handle: cough, rash, headache. With patients I've seen before, if these issues can be handled expeditiously, I catch up on other parts of their lives they've told me a little about in the past: children starting school, dogs put down, mothers-in-law moving in—all the human experience and complexity that makes medical office practice an intimate profession.

With all my patients now, whether or not I've seen them before, I typically ask whether they will have enough money to pay for the medication I prescribe. If they have no medical insurance, whom will they borrow money from? If they have a copay, will they be able to cover it? I want some sense, in advance, if the prescription will never be filled, the medication never taken. These questions sometimes lead to a larger discussion where they offer only a glimpse, the tiniest detail, of their financial situation that reveals the precariousness of their lives outside this office *when they're feeling well*. Some admit to what they will go without in order to fill my prescription: a meal, a bus ride, a birthday gift for a spouse. Some admit to skipping days of medication so they can buy a toothbrush or a window fan.

I grew up comfortably as the child of a high school teacher and a social worker; I worked through college and medical school. By the end of my studies I had some debt, but not too much, only the bills of a young person who had no property or dependents. I knew very little about real-world finances when I started medical school. By the time I finished training in the late 1980s, I could go on about anatomy and physiology, about the beautiful intricacy of the body; I could review its systems and its ailments. I could report on microbes and the immunology of transplantation, but not about the social drivers—poverty among them—that made people stressed and sick and brought them to a doctor's office. I had never taken a course in social services systems or how broken and struggling persons got along in the world outside the hospital. I knew illness but had little perspective on health. There were—and still are—lots of gaps in medical training. Like most young doctors starting to practice medicine on their own in the world, I had no idea what I would actually need to know to make people feel better, physically or emotionally—

the primary job of an office practitioner, no matter what specific medical problem a patient seeks help for.

In the beginning, patients rarely offered information about their finances unless I asked. A decade into practice, when I began to venture beyond how a patient might pay for the medication I'd prescribed and deeper into the topic of finances, I tried to inquire without being too intrusive or judgmental. I understood why most doctors also rarely asked (unless symptoms dictated) about sex or drinking; like money, these were delicate, secret subjects, and why ask unless you had something to offer? But acting gently curious was a way to hear details about a patient's home life that might be relevant to the reason they came to see me and could be important for the lasting effects of any advice or course of medication I was about to offer. Maybe patients' reluctance to answer my more prying questions about money was based on their feeling that it wasn't my business, or that I understood little about their kinds of life problems, what it was like trying to survive in their world. Maybe they were ashamed (as with the details of sex and drinking) or thought that such conversation would lead to my disapproval or a sense of despair. Even when they found themselves discussing their finances with me, they rarely asked for specific help or advice. How could a doctor help?

With each of the twenty-five years I've worked in this office, I've come to know a little bit more about the economics of everyday life for my patients. Patients have taught me a great deal, but it is still less than I need to know: about Temporary Disability Insurance, about dog-racing payouts, about court fines and bail, about car impoundments and pawn shop interest rates and illicit drug prices and evictions. Practicing medicine in my office has been like enrolling in a lifelong course on how people manage to survive against the odds.

Every person who doesn't have enough money has a money story. It's what they think about whenever they aren't worried by that cough, or rash, or hideous headache that has led them to see a doctor. Every doctor knows from experience that people are incredibly resilient, emotionally as well as physically. Sometimes they express distress or rage about their financial situations — *this is what I used to have, this is how far I've fallen* — and other times they laugh about their money problems. What patients tell me is humorous and heartbreaking, irrevocable and hopeless, and their experiences are still very often foreign to me. Their nerves aren't always steady. They want security, less anxiety. They want things beyond their reach. They tease me about the limitations of my role when they tell me they're short on rent: "What are *you* gonna do about it?"

This is what I've done when they've asked: I've helped them draw up monthly household budgets. I'm no expert, but I've looked over income tax forms and double-checked math. I've reviewed cell phone plans. I've wondered aloud who advised them to pay the minimum on credit card bills, allowing the interest to carry forward. When they want my opinion about a community college course they are thinking of taking, I question them about hidden costs, sometimes unintentionally undermining their optimism. I admit when I don't know an answer. I try my best to listen, which is the surest way not to be condescending. They have no financial advisers, no one to tell these secrets to. They rarely — if ever — know anyone who has a lot of money. I've gone home reminding myself adamantly but achingly that I am not accountable for their economic well-being, even when it bears on their physical and emotional health. There is a future I wish I could offer them, but the fantasy of a miracle solution is a trap. Except for those who buy lottery tickets, the folks in my office have given up on magical thinking.

These are people who nervously swivel their eyes and heads expecting the worst — nothing static, everything moving and shifting. They manage despite the fact that there are no comfort zones in these lives. I take courage from their answers.

If you listen to patients one by one, they will tell you something about a society. Since the Great Recession of 2008, I have seen more unemployed patients, more who've been displaced by foreclosure. Medical bills have bankrupted more Americans than any other type of expense. Each of these stories is about feeling broke in some way. I have divided the book into four parts, following the themes patients address and return to again and again: money, home, work, and self. Most patients will appear only once, although Perry's surprising story appears throughout these pages and crosses the four themes. My style is meant to be raw, offering what I hear and the few words I say so that I can learn more. Sometimes the stories are so grim I don't know what to say. I answer clumsily, or not at all.

I am anything but certain, and in my bleaker moments I wonder if in fact I might not be making things worse by suggesting there is some hope. The economics of empathy — who gets it, who deserves it, who is denied it — is complicated and brutal.

Now and then I interrupt their stories in these pages with American facts you may not know or remember but that continue to bother me. They might argue for new policies, or at least a new conversation around poverty. No political candidate or party should be allowed to ignore the subject.

These are not stories of sickness or of bodies, the usual subjects of a doctor's writing. I provide no diagnoses. I present these stories from a doctor's office because perhaps poverty should be approached from a public health perspective, as the moral perspective alone has failed us. They are stories of anguish, of delight despite the storytellers having little, of how people spend their time and cash, and how just getting by might affect their health. Knowing how people manage is part of a doctor's work.

In the end, I hope to give you a view of my neighborhood, and perhaps yours. I've come to understand that even if the street is quiet, the lives in the buildings are seldom easy. The doctor in his office gets only a glimpse. I hear a tiny piece of a story whose completion I may or may not have the energy to think much about at the time, but whose suggestiveness stays with me, moves me, makes me conscious of the closing in and the wearing down in the lives of the poor, and of my own good fortune.

GOOD CHANCE

More than half of the U.S. population will live in poverty at some point before the age of sixty-five.

MONEY

What's Left: Perry

"I'm so broke I have to rinse off paper plates. I'm paid on the first of the month: $723 in social security, $158 in food stamps. My rent is $222, thirty percent of my income, but that includes electricity. The building charges me $11 per month per AC, and I need two—one in the bedroom and one in the den—for my COPD."

It's summer, and Perry's thick finger wipes the sweat from the corners of a mustache that has lost its color but had once been brown. I can see he's not happy with the temperature in my office. He coughs to make the point. He has visits with me every two months, but only today, after a year, when I ask him to tell me about things at home, does he dive into the details.

"I keep an extra freezer, which I pay $6 per month for because I have eighteen grandkids. I keep two $100 bills in a safe and $157 in a checking account. I owe $55 a month on some furniture I bought, a curio with a glass front where I keep pictures of my mother and of my son who died. With anything I have left, I buy food to give away to people in the building whose money runs out before mine does."

Splitting

"We pool all the money. My husband gets $580, same as I get. We both get $199 in food stamps, a little more in the summer. He cuts his father's dog's hair for $50 a month. My son don't work, but his wife gets $780. If she told SSI [supplemental security income] she was married to my son, she'd only get $580. Her daughter gets $520."

"Three bedrooms?" I ask.

"And a parlor," she says. I appreciate her use of such an old-fashioned word.

"What's left after rent, gas, and electric, we split, and my husband gives me $200, which I spend on toilet paper and cleaning supplies and trash bags and dog food. If I had more money, I'd buy me my popcorn, candy, and soda. I like my junk food. Or I'd save for a vacation. I've been on a plane once, thirty years ago to Florida. I didn't like the plane, but I still think fondly of that last vacation."

Won't

"My family was suffering with me gone for work all the time. I couldn't do it anymore. I said to the man I work for, 'What about one or two weekends a month instead of four?' He said, 'That won't work for me. You've put me in a bad spot. I already trained you.' I said, 'I'm willing to compromise.' 'There is no compromise,' he said."

"That puts you in a bad situation," I say.

"I can't go on unemployment—I have no money in there since I'm self-employed. I can't get TDI [temporary disability insurance] because my employer won't sign off that I'm disabled and won't take me back. I can't sleep. I've even tried warm milk. I walk the house, and sleep in other rooms, and my kids ask me why I'm never in my bed in the morning. There's just stress on my brain. I can't think straight.

"I talk to my mother. She's not alive, but talking to her helps."

Child Support

He touches his heavy lower lip, remembering. In the quiet, I notice the room smells of nicotine and dog.

"My son is thirty-seven now. His mother came from a lot of money. I left my son when he was one. My ex-wife didn't want child support, she didn't need it, she owned two apartment buildings. She told me never to worry about her or my son. She didn't ask for alimony.

"I don't talk to her again for years after I leave the state; I never see my son; he never calls me.

"When he's seventeen, he gets into a car accident. He breaks his arm and hand. My ex-wife has three lawyers sue the other driver but loses the case. The lawyers cost a lot, and all of a sudden she wants child support. She'd retired at forty-six, and I don't know what happened to the rest of her money. Anyway, I go into work one day and my boss tells me that the state had called and he had to take money out of my check. That was the first I heard of it. All of a sudden I'm paying $50 a week. And I owe $79,000 in back payments and interest."

"That must have come as a shock," I say. I am aware of our separate and unbridgeable histories.

"I've been paying this now for twenty years. Every year they take my federal tax refund. I didn't have a lawyer to fight any of it.

"Last week I get a call from my ex-wife out of the blue. She tells me my son got married and divorced, but that he's a good boy, a good man. He just bought himself a motorcycle. 'No. *I* bought him a motorcycle,' I tell her. He's my blood, but if I saw him, I'd punch him in the face."

Christmas

"I have jewelry at the pawn shop and pay $8 a month to keep it there, and would need $300 to get it back. It all happened when I bought Christmas presents. I felt bad about signing the temporary custody order and being away, so I bought my daughter presents. She won't get any next year."

Her bright eyes search mine for disapproval.

Giveth and Taketh Away

"I learned only this year that, because I'm on SSI and I *don't* live in subsidized housing, if I file taxes I can get a $350 refund back if I show my rent receipt. No one at SSI told me about this refund for the last five years. So I did it, and I got $350, but the state took it to pay a fine from twelve years ago for driving without a license."

She doesn't seem very disturbed by this turn of events. Her mother usually drives her to appointments.

"Next year, I'll get $350 more and I can then get a driver's license. Of course then I need an SR22, which is license insurance, because I was caught driving without insurance too."

Don't Look Back

"My father and I were thinking of bidding on a foreclosed property. My father had $10,000 saved. I went out to the bakery for an hour, and he called a man he knew for less than twenty-four hours, the real estate man who let us in to look at that property. While I'm still at the bakery, the man came over, and my father gave him the $10,000, but it turns out the house wasn't really available, and now I need a lawyer to try to get the $10,000 back."

I know he has been caring his father since his mother died. He's told me that his father needs so much physical help that he rarely leaves the house. I imagine he'll never leave his father alone to make a bakery run again.

"My father's the type to say, 'If it's done, it's done.' He carries no guilt on him that he lost the money."

Half Smile

"I got all the bottom teeth pulled. That was covered by insurance. But I don't know if dentures to replace them are."

Ends Meeting

She comes in sweating. Even though my office is on a bus route, she's ridden her bicycle eleven miles along the small highway to my office, which is in a generic, four-story glass medical building with windows that don't open on the edge of our spreading city.

"I sell my food stamps to pay for electricity, gas, cat food, and toilet paper. I get 75 cents on the dollar. If you want it bad enough, they'll only pay you 50 cents. Then I go to the food bank with my boyfriend's food stamps and get two bags."

Sometimes I hear their lives as commentaries on my own. She has never eaten in the fashionable places I take my family.

"We eat a lot of eggs, pancakes, home fries, rice. I make $9 per hour, forty hours a week, that's $360. So with taxes I take home a thousand a month.

"We got a new place after his sons threw us out. We owe $750 a month rent, but I'm already behind. Since he wasn't working, I made my boyfriend sell his car. He put it on Craigslist, and we got $500. I gave that right to my landlord. It was his mom's car. He didn't use it. He couldn't afford the insurance or taxes."

DEFINITIONS

The official poverty rate in the United States is determined by comparing a family's pretax cash income to an income poverty threshold. If a family's income falls below this threshold—today $24,000 a year for a family of four— that family is considered to be poor. This threshold was developed in the 1960s and set the poverty line at three times what it cost for the minimum daily food required to satisfy nutritional requirements, because food was then found to account for one-third of the cost of living.

So today that puts about fifteen million children in the United States—21 percent of all children—in families in poverty.

Since the 1960s, the threshold has been adjusted to account for inflation only, despite the fact that food now accounts for only one-seventh of the cost of living, which includes unavoidable expenses such as housing, child care, medicines, and transportation.

Therefore, on average, families need an income of about twice the old threshold to cover basic expenses. Using this standard, 43 percent of children live in poor families.

Most of It: Perry

"I have this woman friend who gives me money. She won $600,000 in the lottery. She hands out $10,000 like it's ten dollars. I take her money, but I'm going to give it back to her."

"Why does she do that?" I ask.

"She's crazy. I keep it in the bank for when she's less crazy and she can have it all back. When I was younger, if it were my money, I'd have spent it drinking. I used to drink a lot because I couldn't relax. I wasn't a bad drunk—I didn't get into car accidents or fights. I still functioned. But I would have spent most of it, maybe all of it."

Someone Else's Problems

"Last year I put all my money into a car. Paid cash for it, $1,200. Then after three months, someone stole it. From right in front of my building. I only had liability insurance. I'd thought about more insurance, but I weighed it out and decided not to."

I have almost no insurance on my car either, I want to tell him. My car's going on 130,000 miles, and if someone wants to steal it, they can have it. But his tone suggests there's more bad news coming.

"Things didn't work out in my favor, I'd say. I called the police, and they got upset with me. There's nothing we can do, they said. It's not a priority. If it pops up, we'll notify you, they said. Pops up? With $800 saved right now, I don't have enough to buy something decent and reliable; $800 only buys someone else's problems."

Knowing the Routine

"My ex-wife embezzled from the Girl Scouts where she was treasurer. It's not clear who called them, but the police asked her to come in. She hired a lawyer and refused to go. The police came to pick her up on an afternoon when my daughter was in the house. They were very professional; they asked my wife to come outside. She called me and asked me to come right over. She told our daughter, 'Mommy did something wrong,' and that there are consequences to one's actions. They took her to the local station where she was arraigned.

"She had to tell her boss, and she lost her job at the bank, but got a job at another bank the next day before the charges showed up on any background check. Once they do the check, they never do it again. She's had several embezzlements in the past, so I've been through this. That's part of why we got divorced."

I'm thinking about what his ex-wife told her daughter, who was eight years old, that day. I remember my sons at eight, how when they cried, their tears rolled as slowly as oil down their beautiful cheeks.

Texting

"I text my best friend Lyn, 'How are you?' And she texts back: 'I'm broke. FML.'"

She surmises from my expression that I don't follow.

"Fuck my life."

I smile.

"I don't answer because I know she's using again and her next text will be: 'Do you have any money?' I used to keep a safe under my bed with about $800, but I gave it to my mother so I wouldn't have to lie to my best friend when she comes over begging."

Car Trouble

"I'm working to get my license back so next time I don't have a get a train ticket from my sister to visit my mother. It was suspended for unpaid tickets. I didn't know it got suspended. But I hadn't driven in a year until last weekend when I took my girl's car out to the store. I got pulled over because a blinker was out."

"That's bad luck," I say.

"The car was impounded. With the court cost, my girl had to pay $697. That's when I learned my license was suspended from not paying the tickets. I'm taking care of that now.

"My girl gives me $10 a month, I go down to the courthouse to pay every month. It takes three buses to get there. All day."

I wonder if he takes the bus here. Amazingly, he's never been late for one of our appointments. In twenty years I've never ridden the bus in my home town.

"But it keeps them off my back. I still owe $250. I'll have to take the driving test again. I owed those tickets for five years. I got six tickets at once on one day driving through New York on my way up from Georgia. I had the wrong plates, no insurance, the car was unregistered, a front light was out, and I had no seat belt. But my license was legit. The cop gave me a break not taking the car away or putting me away. He must have felt bad. We had all our clothes in the car."

Angel Investing

"I get $931 a month, and my subsidized one-bedroom costs $238," she says when I admire her oversized blue cell phone. "I spend $150 on cable, $50 on electric. I bought this $700 phone last month, but it's a really great phone. My real luxuries are the internet games, the MMOs [massively multiplayer online games]—I spend $40–50 a month on that. I meet people from around the world, and even chat with a few of them. *League of Angels* is one where I collect heroes and compete. You have the option to spend money on VIP things, perks that put you ahead of other players, into higher levels."

BULK

A pack of thirty-six rolls of two-ply toilet paper costs around $15, or 42 cents a roll; buying each individually will cost $1. If you don't earn much, you can't afford the higher up-front cost of purchasing in bulk. And if you miss out on sales of larger packages, you have to go out to buy more toilet paper when it runs out and therefore need to visit stores more often, which means more gas, more bus fare.

Checks and Balances

"My father put my name on two of his bank accounts as a co-signer. He did it eight years ago without me knowing it. Why would a bank do that? Aren't they supposed to contact me?

"My father has lived with me for fifteen years, you know, but my niece told him to do it. She was trying to get me in trouble."

I want to hear why she would do that, but I'm not going to interrupt.

"I can't have more than $2,000 in any account because of my SSI—that's one of the rules. SSI sends me a letter six months ago: you owe $43,000. That's when I find out my name has been on his account for eight years.

"I go to the bank and there's my name, but it's not my signature. I go to my niece and tell her that I will sue her if she doesn't confess to forging my name. She says my father forged my name.

"I've never taken any of my father's money. Anyone could see every check for him goes in untouched, and there are no withdrawals in my name. I brought every canceled check to SSI to prove I never used his money, but they tell me I'm lying. They stop sending me my regular monthly check for $800 that I live on and cut off my health benefits. I tell them I'm not giving them a penny, arrest me. Meanwhile, I have to sell my baseball cards to raise some cash."

Workout

"I'll be able to pay my sister back and my girl too. I got a job finally."

"That's some good news," I say.

"I'm the guy who picks things up and puts things down. I open the back gate of the truck and throw down the ramp and pick up the kegs and go down the ramp and into the walk-in refrigerator and pile them up, the new ones on the old ones. Three hundred times a shift. I bring three shirts to work. It's a great workout. I make $411 a week and spend it like an idiot on energy drinks, but I'll be getting out of debt soon, I know."

A Place to Start

"My mother has four doctors — eye, hip, heart, women's stuff. She was bleeding down there. They snipped something off and they still didn't know why she was bleeding. Does that make sense? Isn't that why they snipped it?"

I am thinking of how to reply when she starts again.

"She has no cartilage in her hip and is in terrible pain, but her heart doc says she can't have surgery. She has arthritis everywhere. Her hands are scrunched up. They shut off our electricity because we owe $2,500; heat's $250 a month and we're waiting to have that shut off next.

"She tells me to quit smoking, that'll save us money, but I'm too stressed to quit. I'll quit when I'm less stressed. That'll happen some time. If I were to start to quit, I'd start with the one that I smoke on the way to the bathroom when I wake up to pee. There's *one* cigarette I could quit," she says proudly.

It is difficult to imagine her quitting.

Vandals

"Someone messed with my car. I don't have enough now to pay $79 to get the handle on my door fixed. So I have to get in on the passenger side."

Not How It Looks

"My ex, who makes $90,000, has been asking me for more child support even though I make $20,000. She's vindictive because my daughter loves my new girlfriend, that's all."

He sits like an unexploded bomb, and a feeling of intense fear rolls over me.

"Child Services is backing her because they just want to get more money out of me, that's how they exist, they get paid by the government to get money from men. They couldn't give a shit about the kids. They get bonuses the more they bring in."

Spending

"I called OSHA one day and told them there was a gas leak at work because I had a headache. Another time I sat on the bus thinking I was going to literally explode. I wanted to take my clothes off in the lobby of my apartment building, and the day I actually took them off, I was taken to the hospital."

He always frightens me a little with his wild grin and his anticipation that I might be the one person who properly understands the dangers of the world.

"My check now goes to the mental health center; they are the payee, appointed by the court. They pay my bills. They pay my rent, $425, cable, $108, medication copays, $60. I use my food money, $400 a month, for cigarettes, which is around $300. I save money by eating only PBJs and ham and cheese. My family sometimes helps with my cigarettes. I'd like better food. My dog costs me $150 a month. Cleaning supplies, laundry, $20. I have a cockatiel, Sammy. I have no phone. I don't go to the movies. I wanted a sixty-inch TV, but they blocked it and I got thirty-two inches. I have to spend what I get, that's one of the rules, so I spend my whole life worrying about the money."

Long Waits

"It takes two and a half hours to get to my mother in the nursing home. I take a bus from my house to the airport, then I have to walk an hour from there."

Cursed. More stories of woe. I expect nothing else. He feels trapped in this contingent mode of existence, I understand. Today, like most days, there's no point in encouraging him.

"I didn't go yesterday because I couldn't move my arm after that railing came out and I fell. I tried to put my glasses in my breast pocket and reaching like that set off the pain. I had to go to bed for three hours. I can't use a cane with that arm. I can't go in the MRI, I get claustrophobia, so they can't tell me if my shoulder's bad too. I've tried five times. I never thought I'd be like this. All screwed up and fifty cents to my name."

MADLY DEEPLY POOR

You may be one of the more than three million Americans who live on less than $2 a day. Or you may be one of the more than five million who live on less than $4 a day. That's equivalent to the population of Minnesota. Zero percent of Germany's population is at this level.

Primes: Perry

"I did everything I wanted to do in life. I was in the marines and went around the world. I boxed, heavyweight. I was six foot one, seventy-three inches, 199 pounds. Prime numbers. I was used to getting punched in the face by my father. I was undefeated, 23–0. But I couldn't turn pro because I had an eye injury. Probably happened before I started boxing, because for some reason my father only hit me in the right eye. He hit my mother too, but she went to work at night, so he hit me."

His big arms remain folded, his thumbs pressing hard into the flesh. He has never spoken of this before in all his visits with me. Perhaps he didn't take it for granted that I would listen. I am disgusted by the image of his father repeatedly punching him in the eye. It has always been miraculous to me how people absorb pain and go on.

"I was drinking up all our money back when I was boxing. My wife could keep up with me drinking but could have fun when she wasn't drinking too. She said, 'If you don't quit you'll lose me and the children.' I quit for seven days. One Friday night I went to the bar after work and when I came home they were all gone. She took whatever money there was, and I haven't had much since."

Too Much

"I don't want or like money. I broke up with a girl because she had too much money. She inherited like $500,000. Her life was suddenly all about money, and I didn't care at all. She'd leave $1,000 on the counter to be nice, but I didn't need charity. She kept wanting to pay for dinner."

Capitalism

"You think I ever relied on my $800 check? I flip things. I buy watches from a friend. I don't ask where they're from. Ten Invicta watches, worth $500; I pay $50 and sell for $100. I sell by calling a few people I know. If you know the items could be a little . . . or might be . . . you have to sell to people you trust."

He's a little superstitious. Or used to speaking in code.

"You don't sell them online to strangers. I'm one of the few people you can call at 4 A.M. and I have cash. If you call me then you got a deal. I'm not trying to make a million. Another $600 and I can get by. I flip watches, jewelry, cars, although cars are more work, going to an auction."

Hot Water

"After the lobster season ended in October, I got hired to do a boiler job."

How can he know fishing and heating systems? How did he learn these skills? I feel defeated by a clogged sink, a blown tail light. I am envious. He knows how things work or don't work. But he is probably envious of me, a guy with a regular paycheck and a job that runs four seasons.

"The owner of the building wrote two checks—one for supplies, one for the job—and made both out to my partner. We got paid in advance, $2,800. My partner cashed the checks and disappeared across the country. I went over to explain to the people. 'The checks weren't made out to me,' I said, 'they were to my partner. And I don't have money for the supplies.' But they told me they were pressing charges. I called a lawyer when the cops came to my door looking for me. I turned bail on personal recognizance. The deal was if I paid back the $2,800 the case would be dropped. The lawyer asked, 'You ever hear from the guy again?' I told him, 'It was my father.' The building owner figured we were in cahoots. But I didn't know my father'd do that. He lives in California and must have needed money to get home. He moved there because the IRS was after him in Florida."

Safe

"I work three nights a week cleaning the local elementary school at $10.50 an hour. I can't go over twenty hours a week or I lose my section 8 housing. So I take home about $189 a week, although last week I made $205. My housing is a four-bedroom worth $950, but I don't have to pay a thing. My daughter, who's disabled, gets $733 a month from SSI and $160 in food stamps. I don't trust anyone with her. She's six and she still needs help potty training. She rips off her diapers all day and shits on the floor. You can't force her to do things."

How can you not be furious all the time even though she's your daughter? Autism with all your other burdens? But on her face is an expression that says only: this is what I have to put up with.

"I pay $100 water, $63 electric, $74 gas, car insurance $76, cigarettes $240 a month, dog food $50, and I buy a rat a month for the snake. I spend $100 in gas because I just drive my daughter around all afternoon rather than stay at home with her grunting and not talking and watching me. I need to get away. I bought a battery and alternator this month for $150. I buy my daughter wipes and special detergent; those are expensive."

I wait, watching her. How does she distract herself? Where's the girl's father?

"My son wants me to waitress at the restaurant where he works because he thinks I'd make good money. But I tell him the first person who tells me the food is cold, I'll throw it at them. I'm not ready to be around people, I'm not there yet. I'd rather clean the school on my own all night even if I make less.

"I give $100 to him every month, because he has a safe where he puts some away for my daughter. There's $3,500 there. I can't let the state see it or they'll take her money or make me pay rent. But I need to know she'd be all right if something happened to me."

Necessities

"I'd say we're somewhere between poor and not *that* poor. I get $739 a month, and $250 in food stamps. My father lives with us, and my daughter works two jobs, and there's my grandson. My daughter works in a nursing home recreation department in the day and the kitchen at night and she makes $1,600, and she gets $100 in food stamps for her son. The rent is $800 for a two-bedroom, and I sleep in the living room."

Sometimes these budgets overpower my sense of reality; for a few disturbing seconds I believe that it isn't that hard to get by with so little money.

"I have a savings account with $300. If I had more, I'd buy an air conditioner for the house, and one for my car. Once I pay the bills — car and insurance, that's $800 a month, plus cable, electric, gas — I have maybe $20 left. We use it to eat out. You have to have Chinese once a month."

Revolution: Perry

"My dad started charging me rent when I was sixteen. I had to *pay rent* in the house I grew up in."

This is the father who punched him in the face. But Perry remains more outraged over the rent. I must have an expression that says I'm appalled by it all and allows him to continue.

"Everything revolved around money. He blamed me for spoiling his life because he had to raise me. When I went to friends' houses I couldn't believe it, people sitting around talking. Our meals were silent. I had a younger sister, and she was the only one he liked. He used to say to my mother, 'You screwed up the other one.' My sister was the only one who he paid college tuition for. No one even asked me if I wanted to go. Instead I worked for him in his paint store. When he fired me, he had my sister tell me."

He squinches his eyes to see my reaction. He's a big guy, but his expression is like that of a child about to be punished: unflinching, but ready. I admire that he's trying to remake himself as a man without alcohol, without anger.

Warranty

"I replaced antifreeze with water and the pipes burst. I needed a new engine. I could have bought a new one for $2,500, but I bought one from a car with 130,000 miles for $500 along with a ninety-day warranty. Drove that car like I stole it. Then returned it in under ninety days and got another one."

The First

"The first of the month is the best. I get $773 in my check plus $193 for food stamps. I pay my rent and whatever's left has to last the whole month—tobacco, my son's birthday gift. The time I have extra money I'll get a haircut," she says. "I haven't had one in six months. Not a color though—I can do that myself. And new sneakers."

Insurance

"My sister's husband was thirty when he flipped his Camaro at 2:30 in the morning and skidded into a tree. I always thought he was a smart guy. He had a big job at Bank of America. But he thought he was sixteen years old. His life insurance company didn't want to pay because they said at an alcohol level of .40 he was trying to kill himself. They called it suicide so they could get out of paying $4.3 million. His case went all the way to the state supreme court, whether that much drinking could be ruled a suicide, and my sister lost after nine years in the courts. Not a penny. When they announced the verdict, his drinking that night was all over the front pages. My sister was never the same."

Barter

"I get $200 for every two weeks of work at the orchard my uncle owns out in the country. We press cider, clean up brush, clean the coolers. I work three farmers markets on Saturdays. I pay $400 a month to my mom for rent, $73 per week in child support ($10 is arrears pay). I roll my own cigarettes, which costs only $20 a week. I trade apples for food."

No Call Back

"About three years ago I was in training for a job at Dunkin, but I couldn't do it. I got a severe migraine from the lights. I applied for SSI for the headaches and seizures and PTSD and high blood pressure, but I missed the phone call because I was fighting with my mother and never called back. So I don't get SSI, only food stamps, $194 a month."

If I could open one of the reflective windows facing the highway, loose papers and despair would fly out from her bag.

Running Tab

"I don't mind going to the hospital. I usually go to the hospital because I don't eat right. I do without. I skip at least one meal a day. When I don't eat breakfast, I eat more for lunch and it messes with the sugar level, you know? I stay in the hospital as long as I can. At least there I eat properly and I don't pay. I just add it to my tab," he says. "I have $100,000 in health care bills since I lost my foot to diabetes. I haven't been paying on those bills. I can't even understand the letters they send with all their red marks. I don't have credit, but I don't borrow either."

EXTINCT

Thirty years ago, for every 100 families with children and no way to pay for basic needs, 68 received federal assistance to help pay bills. Today, it's 23 out of 100.

That's 9 million citizens with zero cash income who still need cash for laundry detergent, toothpaste, and toilet paper (also rent and utilities).

Extinction is the state or process of a species, family, or maybe a federal program, disappearing.

HOME

PRIORITY

In New York City roughly half a million
people are on the list of those seeking
subsidized housing for the 175,000
apartments available to low-income
tenants.

About 5,000 apartments free up annually.

So overall, you have less than a one in a
hundred chance of getting a place.

But if you need a two-bedroom (there are
more of these), you need to have a job
(so you can contribute more to the rent),
or survive domestic violence, so you can
get priority.

Either: Perry

"After boxing, my mind was like a vase that's been dropped and glued, dropped and glued. I was never good with money. My mother wanted me to have at least one decent outfit, and I didn't even have that. She saw the way I dressed and said I was too scruffy."

He's still scruffy. Thick mustache and hair in his eyes that he has to keep pushing aside. Flannel shirts and jeans at every visit. Moccasins he can slip on without bending over. He used to lose himself in physical conflict and tests of endurance, but now he sits extremely still. The back pain and blood thinners for the clots in his big calves have made him introspective. I understand that his swollen legs make it difficult for him to stand for long, and I don't imagine him as a man who enjoys sitting.

"When I left home at twenty, I tried to be all the things she wasn't and hung with the wrong people.

"Now I'm sixty and my sister's had the same job for thirty years and writes poetry. My mother has ovarian cancer. She had to spend all her money to qualify for insurance to keep the treatment going. The chemo doesn't agree with her, but I never did either. All the money I don't have, she doesn't have now either."

Dream House

"I'm forty-five years old and I live with my dad. My dream is to own a house. My credit score is good, but my income's not high, $769 a month. I need to get back to work. The last time was ten years ago when I was a cashier. I'm on disability from my legs, but I'd rather not take the money. How much can a person sit around? How many times a day do I need to clean my house? I'm not like that; it's driving me crazy."

"Have you started looking for a job?" I ask. I try to rid my voice of expectation, which could make her feel worse.

"Maybe I'll be a phlebotomist. They make good money, $20 an hour in the hospital, $35 if you go to people's houses like a visiting nurse. A friend of mind who's a nurse thinks I'd be good. I can stand the sight of blood; it don't bother me. I need to save $600 for the eight-week course. My left leg still swells when I'm on my feet too much, after like three hours. But the lady who draws my blood gets to sit down between patients or when she's writing out labels. I always wanted my own house. There's not a lot of time left for me. In another ten years I'll be too old to take care of a house."

Ransom

"My husband took a restraining order out on me when I went to detox. I came home and he wouldn't let me in. He called the cops and they came over and showed me the order. He claimed he was afraid of me, him 280 pounds, me 120."

When I look into her small bright eyes and hear that she retains a sense of the ridiculous, I have no reason not to believe her.

"Two months later we're in court, both of us without lawyers. The judge has no proof that I'm a threat to him or our daughter but won't let me in the house that has my name on the lease. The judge says come back in three months with a lawyer.

"As we're leaving court my husband says, 'If you sign this temporary custody form you can come home.' My daughter's been calling me every day for months, 'Mommy, come home, when are you coming home?' So, like an idiot, I sign. He doesn't want my daughter, he wants her check. The 620 bucks a month that was half of my disability payment is now in his name."

An Education

She always stands when she talks to me, as if she's ready to bolt.

"I was going to take two courses at the community college. I found out the books for one are $18, for the other $80. Since I withdrew last semester when I went to detox, they took away my financial aid for books. It doesn't make sense. They'll pay thousands for tuition, but not the $98 for the books. So now I can't take the classes and I withdrew again."

Another Story

"My wife, we're legally separated, she falls in a pothole and breaks both her ankles. Hospital, rehab, home. She gets a settlement from the city, and her landlord wants to raise her rent so she moves out, wants to stay with me while she looks for another place.

"I tell her, 'This is my place.' But the second day she's there, she starts rearranging things. It's bad enough that she takes half my closet. I say, 'You can visit, but you need to go home.' I didn't mind her visiting for a weekend, but this everyday stuff is not good. It's been ten years since we lived together. Now she wants to run stuff. She's hardheaded. I say, 'You ain't gonna change me.' She's one of those who ask me what I want for breakfast and then brings me what *she* wants."

I feel aggrieved on his behalf.

"'You move in and don't pay, fine, but don't think you can freeload here for long,' I tell her. 'If you want to pay half, then we can talk.' I say, 'You *do* remember why you left in the first place? You put me in jail, that's why.' That's another story."

Electricity

"I'm glad I have a daughter, but I wish I never met the clown I had her with. Now I'm stuck with him, this man who took a restraining order out on me. It's bad."

She's been seeing me often for her asthma these last few months since she's been back with her husband and taken the house-cleaning job. She admits to overusing the inhaler when she's nervous and running out early, unable to afford a refill. She enjoys telling stories on herself, even the bad ones.

"We live in a three-family house. The man on the third floor pays part of our electric bill because of crossed wires; we get charged for his use. He gives my husband money every month. Yesterday he texts my husband to tell him he left money outside our door where I keep my cleaning supplies, but when my husband checks, the money's not there. 'I know you found it,' my husband says to me, 'under your broom.' 'I didn't see it,' I say. 'You're a liar. A sneak. I know you got it. I should punch you.' 'I didn't find your money. I don't have it,' I say. Then I cook him dinner."

Just How It Goes

"My sister-in-law comes over last weekend and says, 'Can you watch the kids, I'll be back in an hour.' She's back in five hours. The kids are three, five, and ten. They sit on my game system for a while, but I only have one game, and they got tired of playing it. She's a junky. I'd never leave her alone in the house. I was raised different. I had no problem with addicts, but they knew not to come around, and if they did, they had to show themselves out. If a neighbor gets high in my building now, I think, do what you want. But don't slam the doors at 2 A.M. I talk to the landlord, who doesn't live there and is an alcoholic. The addicts drink with him.

"The landlord blames us when there's a problem because we're the oldest people there. He blames us for the time when they had to shut the water off in the building and everyone's told not to flush a toilet and someone does, not us, and the pipes break. We're not even home when that happens. Me and the landlord get into an argument. It starts with emotion and ends with money."

I wonder if any of my patients know that I live in a house. Do they know anyone other than me who lives in a house? There is nothing in his way of life I recognize from my own life.

Custody

"I don't like my husband. We don't get along. I don't have the money to move out. We live in the same house but stay in different rooms. We have sex. He'd be even more of a jerk if we didn't."

After all the nasty things she's said about the guy, I'm surprised to hear about the sex, but maybe I shouldn't be.

"I eat dinner with my daughter, but he eats later, although he eats my food. I do his laundry. If I don't, he can be very ugly. I try to go out alone, but he sends my daughter with me. I'd like to go on dates, but that won't work.

"I've relapsed since she was born, which means I might have trouble if I ever tried to get custody back. He's never relapsed. He loves the situation. With me trapped, he can be a jerk when he wants to be. I could leave and find a nice guy, but I won't leave my daughter with him. He wouldn't want to be bothered taking care of her, but he wants to control me. I beg my mother to let me borrow some money to get out, to get my own place, but she claims she don't have none."

I am a giver of small gifts. I can offer her respect, but not safety or a cash advance.

Happy Ending

"The day after my son died, I worked thirteen hours, showered, went to a bar to get drunk, came home, went to sleep, and when I got up, I left for Florida with $300. I didn't know a person there.

"I slept in the Greyhound station and looked for work. I joined this temp agency—construction, cleaning septic tanks—and lived in a trailer with other guys in the agency. When I got into cocaine and ecstasy, I lost my job and lost my place. I bought a tent and lived behind a supermarket in the woods. I'd work now and then, and get a hotel room to shower. I started selling pills as a middle man until I went to jail for three months for missing court dates on drug charges. When I got out, I went back to my tent and I got held up at knife point."

His voice is not urgent; his expression is slack; maybe this is how a person is when, barely past his teenage years, his infant son dies.

"My mom wired me $90, I moved here, met this girl, and I been with her for ten years. Our daughter's nine now."

Meal Plan

"People don't know how to shop. I've mastered how to live on $155 a month. I can get twenty-five pounds of chicken thighs for $40. I fill up my freezer and eat them every meal over a month with black rice, pasta, apples, pineapples, and avocado. But if I eat out, I might meet a girl."

HUNGRY

If last month you were out of money, out of food, and forced to miss meals or seek assistance to feed yourself, you're one of thirty-three million adults or seventeen million children. You're probably deficient in vitamin A, magnesium, and protein. When you eat, you're far more likely to consume starch and refined sugar.

Brought Back: Perry

"I'm in the car, maybe six years old, and we're in this lumber yard, stealing lumber. I could tell we were doing something wrong the way my father was looking around. I was afraid we'd be caught.

"Another time we came home and the TV was gone, the furniture was gone. As a child you're afraid someone was in your house. It turns out that he had the house broken into for the insurance money. Three weeks later our things were brought back."

He speaks loudly. His stomach wobbles under his shirt; he is fifty pounds off his boxing weight. He's a large man. Fifty years later, his father is still chasing him.

Family Ties

"Went home last week. Had to. It's my mother. She's all alone there with my handicapped brother."

He takes a deep breath, nods once, looks me in the eye. He wants to be sure I understand what loyalty means to him.

"When she gets sick, all of us get together and take turns. My mom don't ask for help. She don't like to be catered to. My brother, he's twenty-four, who's handicapped, he's like a child, he don't really talk that well. He can't be on his own. Doesn't wipe himself right. He's out of the house during the day at this work program. They teach him life skills. He puts things in boxes — toys, hygiene products — for companies. My sister paid for my ticket. But I don't see how I can pay her back."

Phones

"I find my son on Facebook in June. I last saw him ten years ago when he was fifteen, when he was living with his father. Before then he was living with me, but I couldn't get day care and I didn't want to go on welfare, so I sent him to live with his father in another state. I knew his grandmother, his father's mother, loved him to death and nothing bad would happen to him. I saw him until I didn't have a car, and then it was hard to get there. His father told him I never called.

"In June I found out he was homeless. He tells me on Facebook he goes from here to there, he doesn't like being called homeless. He says he has a roof over his head. He has giant holes in his ear lobes in the picture. I send him a phone."

She's gripping the oversized blue phone that she never puts down when she's with me for her diabetes check-in.

"That one disappears and I send him another. In July I hear he's in jail for shoplifting. I find out it's the eleventh time in jail for the same thing. It's expensive for him to call from jail, $1.25 a minute. He gets out of jail and decides not to move away. He puts on Facebook: 'Send me money. Buy me a phone.' But he doesn't want to see me. I send him $20 so he can buy another phone, but I see on Facebook he's bought new plugs for his ear holes with the money. That's when I decide I should buy myself a really new phone, a luxury, $700."

Secret

"My older cousin would do drugs in front of me when I was five years old. I'd be on her lap and she'd take out her mirror with its razor blade and lines, and she'd tell me to look away. When I was a little older, maybe eight, she used to breathe pot smoke into a plastic bag and put it over my head, and I must have been a little high because she'd tell me there were silver dollars in her shoes and she'd have me walk over to get them, and she'd say, 'Not there, the other shoes.' And I'd walk across the room to the other pair, and she'd say, 'Not there,' and have me walk back again, and I did this back and forth for a while with her laughing; only a high person would do that."

Her face is flushed when she tells me this.

"Today I only own the one pair of shoes I'm wearing."

Two Possibilities

"My daughter says to me, 'I think I'm bipolar.' I am; her grandfather was. When I was first married, I used to tell my husband I was going out for cigarettes and drove two states over, six hours, to buy a pack. He said, 'That's not normal,' but I thought it was perfectly normal back then, before I started taking medication. My daughter's eighteen. She pays for her own community college and she worries about money."

"What do you worry about for her?" I ask.

"She started going to bed at three in the afternoon this summer, not waking up until the next morning. I thought she was depressed. This week, she's staying at my house and I wake up to use the bathroom and I find her at 3 A.M. on her cell phone playing a game. She's been up for three days in a row, she tells me. She may be bipolar, but she may just be eighteen and stressed out over her bills. Who isn't?"

Business Partner

"When I was fourteen, my aunt let me have drinking parties at her house with my friends, and supplied the alcohol."

And maybe that explains why you still drink a lot? And maybe that explains why you've never really been able to hold a job? I see her as affable and capable, and sadly immobilized.

"At least she spent time with me, and was glad to see me, unlike my mother. The parties stopped for a few years when she got sober. But then when I was in my early twenties, she needed extra money when her daughter, my cousin, had a baby and was living with her. It started with the leftover Percocet after the cesarean. 'You know anyone who wants to buy pills?' my aunt asked me.

"I thought I'd tell everyone about this when she died. But when she actually died, I didn't. She wasn't there to defend herself."

Roomie

"Doc, I divorced two years ago, and the money is not coming in. I get a check for $750 a month and the rent is $600. I need a cell phone. I get food stamps for $196. I don't spend much on food; I'm trying to lose weight anyway using those TV dinners."

She's not making much progress on her weight; her frozen food protocol is not likely to do the job. Most visits she tells me her metabolism is slower than other people's. Some patients call me by last name without the Doctor, some just use my first name, others call me Doc. I don't mind any of these options.

"My son Frankie lived with me and did not want to help with the rent. He got a good job now too, making money. Twenty-two-year-old spoiled little kid. He took two-hour showers. He wanted to keep the heat high to eighty in the house. I asked him for half the rent, but he wanted to spend his money on sneakers. He wanted me to take care of him. Buy all the food, cook it. I said, You gotta go. Even his older brother told me, He's gotta go — don't worry about him. I told Frankie, Grow up.

"Now he's living alone, paying $700 rent, but in a few months when the bills stack up, he'll come running to mommy. Come and apologize, I'll say, and we'll be set."

Second Generation

"My son goes to help his grandmother who has Alzheimer's. Not the kind where you have to clean up after her, the kind where she wants to serve breakfast at 7 P.M. Her husband's there too, although he's been falling and the family finally understood that he'd been drinking. At age seventy-five he's been in and out of detox five times this year. Anyway, my son goes over there to help. That's a lot to handle. Why does he have to take care of his grandparents when they have five children? His aunts and uncles should pay him for doing their work."

She's outraged for her son, and I'm sure she's asked her relatives to pay him, but I can tell that each request is a long, tiring campaign for her.

Separation

"I live alone. I don't want no friends. They talk too much. They'll tell my business if I let them know it. Can't nobody tell me nothing. I don't listen. The only friend I got is my wife. She don't live with me."

He says this not unhappily, maybe proudly.

"I get $950 a month and I spend $280 of it on a car loan for her, which is $10 more than I spend on my rent. We're separated, but I bought it for her when she went back to college at night. She work in the food service, salads, at the college. I talk to her every day about a bunch of nothing, but every day, at 5 A.M. when she go to work, and 3 P.M. when she head home, she calls me from that car. When I really need to talk to her she pick me up when she gets out of work and we go riding for an hour or so."

Shit List

"In my case, I fell. The railing on the front steps came out of the ground, and I broke my arm. I started getting doctor bills. I called the building manager for their insurance company name so I could hand in the bills. I got no answer. He never called back, so I ended up having to call a lawyer."

He's begun to see himself as cursed.

"But I realize they will throw me out if I sue the housing authority. My ex-wife got electrocuted putting in a plug in her apartment in the building. Her fingers turned black. They eventually gave her $1,400, but they made it rough for her. They'd give her notices on bogus stuff. You weren't allowed to smoke a certain distance from the building, four feet from the property line, and they wrote her up for smoking too close. You get a few of those and they get rid of you. You get on their shit list.

"Even if I got $10,000 in a settlement, they'd turn me out. Then I'd have to go on a list. It would take forever to get another place. Everyone in the building is already trying to get out; my neighbor is no. 432 on the list. I didn't realize it until I became one, but there are a lot of poor people out there."

What's Real

"I feel demonic activity going on. I've been seeing things, or I might be seeing them. I'm being sabotaged. The police department won't drop the case against me though they know I'm innocent. They showed up because I asked for a lie detector test. They have keys to my building."

Whenever I see him, I remember his story of taking his clothes off in the lobby of his building. He's attuned to disrespect, so I always roll my chair toward him as he speaks as a signal of interest.

"There's drug traffic in the building. Johnny, he's 110 pounds, a mess. He doesn't even live in the building, his mother does. He's just no good. I cursed him out for leaving the door open. I told him how I feel. He called the cops on me, but he can get away with it because he's an informant. He tells them that I'm harassing him. He cut himself and made himself bleed and blamed me. The proprietor and the police know he's lying. But I open my mouth and they arrest me overnight. I'm released in less than twenty-four hours. They know I'm poor and have no power and they can fuck around with me. It would be over if I had a real lawyer."

Don't Ask, Don't Tell

"I'm not an elaborate person. I'm satisfied with the way I live. These pants are thirty years old, this shirt over ten years old. But right now I'm totally broke. I got only change in my pocket. I could have used some of the money I might have gotten from that broken railing."

Something has happened; he had not expected it; he doesn't understand it at all. I think he's surprised that I let him complain about his life.

"It began after my mother got sick. She costs me now. I need to pay her life insurance, that's $30 a month, her health insurance is $30 a month, I don't know why I pay that since she's eighty-eight years old. She needs diapers and soap; for some reason they don't get her diapers at the nursing home; they wrap her in blue chucks. She gets $956 but pays the nursing home $892 a month. The woman has been an angel her entire life, so it's okay if I have to live on an English muffin a day. I'll get a check on the first, five days from now.

"I'd never borrow. If my kids knew I didn't have, they'd give to me, but that would kill me. Thank God they're each doing something wrong and they don't come around—the youngest one with his DUI bracelet, my daughter with her addict boyfriend and new baby, the oldest one with a wife who's always been against me."

TIRED

Six hours of sleep is a healthy amount. If you are below the poverty line you are far less likely to get six hours regularly than someone who earns more. Why? Maybe you wake up earlier for a longer commute. Maybe you have multiple jobs. Maybe there's more noise in your neighborhood. You're more likely to be in pain. Maybe you are afraid of someone breaking in. It's more likely that someone's ill in the house. Maybe you're waiting for child support or a SNAP check or a disability payment.

Reach: Perry

"My mother once broke a wooden spoon over my head. After that, when she was angry, she went for plastic, which didn't break. When I got bigger and could avoid her, she tied a string to a plastic spoon to get more reach."

The first evasive moves of a boxer. He giggles, although he's trained himself to keep his mouth closed when he smiles so no one can see that he's missing teeth. He is always on his best behavior around me, trying to add warmth, or at least take away the roughness that has surrounded him his whole life.

"I love women, but I think of money problems the same way, always coming after you."

Marriage

"Between me and my husband it's no good. That man gave me trouble all the years we've been married. He's seventy now and took over his father's body. He's his father's twin. He took his attitude too.

"I told him I want a separation, and this is his answer, 'Why the hell would you want to do that? You're old. How long you gonna last, five years?' 'I'm in better shape than you,' I say. 'I got things to do.' He says, 'You hate my guts.' 'I never said that,' I tell him. 'You still can't have any of my money,' he says.

"Here are my reasons for leaving."

"Tell me," I say, although there'd be no stopping her, really.

"I never wanted to be in that house. His brother talked him into buying it, and I never liked it. It still needs fixing after forty-three years. I never liked the kitchen. I wanted a single level that was finished, not a work in progress. The second reason is that my mother follows me around the house. She lived with us, and died there, in my arms, and now I constantly think about her, and I want to get away from her. The third reason is that I want to get away from him. But when I ask for five bucks for gas, he asks me why he should give it to me."

Boys

"I had three boys, and two jobs, and I was doing drugs. But I was strict. I'd send them to their rooms. My oldest says they were so scared of me when I walked by. I was old school. I slapped but never used my fist. I never beat them, made them black and blue. I wish I could take some of it back."

I believe him. A sense of his humiliation leaps out at me.

"The oldest says he started at age thirty-three, on his birthday. He was living with me after his divorce. He always had shoulder pain; he had two operations. I don't know how he got into heroin, but I saw the signs. He would tell me someone was just dropping him off cigarettes. 'What do you take me for?' I asked him. I went through his drawers. I didn't give a shit; it was my house.

"I take him every morning to methadone. I had to wake him at first, but now I try to make him get up on his own. 'You had the money for drugs, now you can pay for this,' I tell him. He knows he can count on me for the ride, though."

I wonder when he thinks he was thrown off course or if this is the place at which he was expecting to arrive.

Why

"A good friend of mine just killed himself. A guy I used to walk my dog with in the mornings."

"I'm sorry to hear it," I say. "Tell me about him."

"Two days ago, he didn't show up with his dog. His wife came over an hour or two later and asked, 'You seen my husband?' I told her I hadn't, and the next day I hear he hung himself in his garage. He was sixty. He had a wife and a nine-year-old daughter. He seemed as happy as could be the last time I saw him. If anyone complained on that walk, it was me. He had a mutt like mine. I can't understand it. He didn't owe anyone a dime."

Revenge

"When I come in the door from meeting my twenty-eight-year-old daughter who I haven't seen since she was six months old, my new wife says, 'Did you bring me a gift?' 'A what?' 'A souvenir, from your trip.' 'No, I didn't.' 'I'm your wife. The most important person in your life.' 'You are,' I say, 'but why are you coming after me now?' 'You didn't bring me a thing.' 'Get out of this room,' I say, and shut the door on her.

"Next thing, the police are there. They take me away, saying she claims I hit her. I'm in jail for one night. I miss the first game of the World Series. I go to court the next day and the judge releases me, since there's no evidence. But there's an automatic no contact order."

How does this happen to people? What part is he not telling me?

"I go to the store to get some big black garbage bags to take my stuff out of that apartment. I call the police, because I can't go over there without them, because of the no contact. I stop in the building manager's office, with the police, to tell him I'm getting my things. He says, 'Her name isn't on the lease, yours is. She has to leave, not you.' The police say, 'We better tell her that news while you wait outside in the hall.'

"We go upstairs and she started performing for them, crying, falling to the floor. I tell them to tell her I'll be back in two days. When I get back, she's cleared the place out, even the toilet paper."

No Escape

"My brother abused me. He was fifteen when it started; I was six. I was eleven when I told my mother and father. They didn't help me. Finally, I told at school and I was sent to foster care."

He's avoided talking about this with me for four years. This is the first time. I remind myself that he wants something from me, as all of my patients do. They come here with the purpose of being recognized.

"I'd see my biological family, including my brother, at family events over the years. When I was thirty-five, I needed money to help take care of my kids after my wife left me and left town. I went to my brother and asked him for $100. He refused. 'After what you did to me, it's the least you can do,' I said. I threw an ashtray and hit my brother in the head and left him stunned on the floor. I took his money and his car. He called the police. They found me thirty minutes later, red-handed. My brother just wanted the money back, but the police pressed charges for armed robbery. I went to jail for two years. My kids went into foster care."

Hospitality

I can tell whatever's coming next, he needs to get off his chest.

"The manager had a key to my apartment. He let himself in and when I came home he was watching my TV and had fixed himself a drink. 'I can get you for breaking and entering,' I said. If I told his boss, he'd have been fired on the spot, but then I wouldn't get a break on the rent. Instead I called his girlfriend. His girlfriend said, 'I'm done with him.'

"When I was on the phone, he poked my head with one finger. My mother used to slap me behind the head when she drank. He poked me and reflexively I punched him and broke his glasses. 'You'll pay for that,' he said. 'Do it again and I'll kill you,' I said. 'Thanks for the hospitality,' he said."

The Old Ways

"We have the cooler for the months we can't pay the electricity. Ice is three bucks for ten pounds, but it lasts almost a week. At least the food keeps pretty good. If I owned my own place and couldn't afford a refrigerator, I'd be fine with ice."

The Next Generation

"I'm such a fuckup. But my older kids aren't. Jesse works for a landscaper. He saves money. He's getting married. Dennis is twenty-one and came in third in a hip-hop contest. He raps about posterity and the laws of attraction. He raps to kids with cancer in the children's hospital. He works eleven to eleven as a busser. When he was little, I thought I'd kill him, but now he's amazing. I *did* that, I think, looking at him; I raised him right. I made sure he opened doors for ladies and never put his hands on them. Every night at five we ate dinner at the table. None of that ever happened for me. I had to learn it off TV. I taught my kids that money is replaceable, but they should still put it in the bank."

The Other Half: Perry

"Before all the talk about the 1 percent, people on TV used to talk about the 'other half.' How the 'other half' lives. But I think of the other half as the second half of the month. That's the only time some of my neighbors visit me. They come to me for coffee filters and sugar and sometimes bread. Always after the 15th."

He speaks somberly, but I can tell he's proud that they come to him. A feeling of identification stirs when I look at him. Why do I think of *him* after he leaves the office? What sets him apart? His kindness, his willfulness, his melancholy?

"They get bigger checks than I do; how do they run out of money in the middle of the month? They eat out or do take-out. I see the pizza delivery guy here every day until the 15th. Then they come knocking."

Survival Benefits

"Jimmy Jr. gets $400 a month in survival benefits from his mother. He's handicapped with CP [cerebral palsy]. She was a nut; there were a lot of things wrong with her, maybe bipolar; she'd go off and smash her husband with a meat grinder. She collapsed and died in front of Jimmy Jr. when he was four. She'd told me the week before, 'I'm not gonna make it to forty.' I said, 'Don't talk like that.' She said, 'I'm going to die, and when I do, will you take care of my son for me?' I'm not thinking nothing of it because she was very off the wall. And then she died. I married her husband. Now Jimmy Jr.'s mine and his $400 is what I live on."

Two-Family

"My boyfriend was living in the apartment downstairs in his father's two-family house. Then his father died and his father's second wife was living there, until she went to assisted living. My boyfriend, the only son, became the owner of the building. We're living there and we can make it because I have a job on the last shift at Burger King and my boyfriend has food stamps."

"You're careful with your money," I say. But what do I know? My life largely involves *not* thinking much about money as I replace deck planks, buy new rugs, refurbish a kitchen. I should give more money to charity than I do.

"At some point, I don't know why, he signed the house over to his two kids, who were twenty-four and twenty-six. He spoiled those two boys—bought them ATVs, bought them their first cars. One day, a realtor comes into our apartment with this couple. That's how my boyfriend finds out that his sons are selling the house and we've got to move out in three weeks. He doesn't even get mad, he loves those boys so much. They sell it and each buys a house of his own."

Romance

"It was February 29th and supposedly that's some special day when women can propose to men. She wanted to get married, and I said, 'Okay, why not?'"

"Congratulations," I say.

"It doesn't matter. It's nothing. Sixteen years we've been going together and I don't even live with her. I'm done with other women; I'm fifty-five years old, women don't look at me. I'm gray. We were both writing wills. She had a pension, I had a pension. She said, 'I want it to go to you.' She said, 'We got to get the rings. We should pick them out together.' I said, 'No, you should just go and get two bands.' I went to a store on my lunch break and got my finger measured. She ordered the rings online and they arrived in the mail. I said, 'How about a justice of the peace?' She knew a chapel. It was the one she got married in before. I said, to my son, 'What are you doing next week? Want to be my best man?'"

Moving Again

"We've been there three months and my landlord raised the rent, so we have to move again. He told me when I moved in he would raise the rent every year, but then he raised it $75 to $825 this month."

There's a finality to her tone. This just isn't fair is all I can think.

"There's a deck in the back that's rotted and I told him to fix it, someone would get hurt," she says. "Then last week I stepped on a broken stair and fell through. My back went numb and I called the ambulance. He was worried I would sue, but he still told me to get out by the end of the month. The man who lives downstairs told me the landlord wants someone like him with housing assistance in my place so he can put the rent up and have it guaranteed. He probably thinks he can get $1,000 for mine; the state will pay $1,000.

"I thought I found another place around the corner, then the lady changed her mind."

Not the Same

"I paid for three sets of braces for my kids. Every cent I had went to those, and I couldn't afford to go to a dentist myself. I brushed twice every day, but my teeth started to go bad. Then my front teeth went and I got partials, but I still had some in the back left. I chewed on one side for three years. About a year ago, I was losing half a tooth a week; they just broke into pieces. Ten months ago, I let them take all my teeth, the ones that were left, seventeen at once."

I wince and moan indiscreetly. "I'm afraid of all dentists," I say.

"They made me top and bottom dentures, but the bottom ones hurt. Now I don't use the bottoms. No one really notices. I don't have a girlfriend so I don't worry about her seeing. At home, I take all my dentures out. I cut things small so I can eat. My favorite thing in the world in late summer was a tomato and cheese sandwich on white bread, but now I'd have to cut and suck it and it's no good like that. It's just not the same."

A Series of Events

"My mom picked up my two dogs because I had no money to pay for their food. I usually don't have much to do with my mother.

"She took them to her house and brought only one back a week later. And the second leash.

"When she came in, I saw she didn't have the puppy. 'Where is she?' I asked. 'You turned on me,' she said. 'How's that?' I asked. 'Because you're still seeing her.' She didn't like the girl I was with. 'I want my other dog back,' I said.

"She went to the police station and told them I'd swung at her."

"Did you?" I ask.

He emits a deep sigh.

"They arrested me.

"They kept me in jail for thirty days because if I fought it they said I could catch up to a year.

"While I was in there I didn't pay my rent, and now I have to move out."

The Secret Lives of Houses

"My mother and I are losing the house my father built. My footprint is in the cement of the foundation. Beautiful triangle windows, sky lights, and big wide oak stairs."

An optimistic smile has always seemed to be his fixed expression, but now he looks confused.

"My father made his money in the car wash business. He cleared $20,000 a month, cash. After he died, my mother started gambling and I started using drugs. We couldn't pay the loan on the house. We're moving out in sixty days."

I have the impulse to give him the loan money. See if he can make a go of his tree work and yard maintenance business. His enthusiasm has always made me root for him.

"We know everything that's wrong with the house after thirty years—the double-paned front window that's about the fall out, the termites, the bad wiring where when you turn on the light in the kitchen, the fan in the bathroom goes on. Someone else will have to pay for the repairs."

NO PLACE TO GO

If you are one of the 1,800 street-faring people living in the Los Angeles neighborhood known as Skid Row, you have the use of one of nine toilets at night. This ratio violates sanitation standards that the United Nations High Commissioner sets for refugee camps.

WORK

LENDERS

You need $200. They will give you $200 cash, and you will write them a check that is postdated for $225. For two weeks, you are paying $25 interest on $200. If you paid $25 on $200 for a year, it would be a 12 percent interest rate, but when you do it for two weeks and then you don't pay it off, and you do another one for the next two weeks, then you do another one for the next two weeks, and you keep this up for a year, it's 800 percent a year.

Work More

"Some days I make $300, some days $100. I need a thousand a week to catch up, so I should be working six days, weather permitting. I need a day off to rest, though.

"My rent is $900 a month, child support $400 plus $100 medical, which I'm $8,800 behind on. I was audited by the IRS a few years ago and couldn't prove that my daughter lived with me and not her mother, so I owe them $5,000. I owe my father $3,800 for the boat motor. I pay $300 a month for the Harley loan, with about $6,000 left, but I'll own that soon. I don't drive it, so I don't pay the $90 a month in insurance. I pay my truck insurance, $150 a month, cable, phone, electric $100 each. I pay $25 a month on my credit card, I only owe $500 there, but I know I should pay that off. Three hundred in cigarettes, $300 in booze, five bucks a day for coffee. Food maybe $200 a month—I live on eggs and potatoes. The answer is I should work more. I miss too many days."

I feel a curious tenderness for him because I've known for years how hard he works. He's decided to say out loud the numbers that must be constantly running through his mind. It's as if I've chanced on a secret door to his planning nature that he keeps hidden from most people.

Bad Business

"I was stabbed right under my ribs by a guy I knew ten years ago at AA. I'd been working on the guy's ex-wife's car at my shop. I returned the car to her, she'd paid, and the ex-husband came in to dispute the bill. I told him it was none of his business and asked him to leave. He left, but a little later, when I'm shutting down the garage, the guy reappeared. He comes toward me, we lock up a little, and I'm stabbed."

"Stabbed," I repeat, still astounded. I wonder if the stabber was drunk.

"I went to the ER, got sewn up, and admitted overnight for a few doses of antibiotics.

"I shouldn't have called the cops. They came, and for some reason they called the building inspector, and he came and my garage got shut down. I never get a break."

Tastes

"Last night we brought in 800 pounds of mantis shrimp. I've never seen one sold in a store. My boss sells them for $7 a pound, right on the dock to the Chinese who buy them as aphrodisiacs. We keep them alive in tanks on the boat. We take them off the mud on the bottom from August to October. I never ate one even though they're free. I couldn't tell you what they taste like. They look like cockroaches."

A Little Extra

"I began prostituting when I was shooting dope. I had a habit that cost me about $80 a day. When I stopped using, I stopped prostituting.

"But I've kept three guys for the last twenty-five years for a little extra money. I kept the three best — they had brains and held jobs and were nice and considerate. Two owned summer houses; one, I think, worked for the state. I see them each once a week. I never say the amount, I guess it's usually around $50 or $100 each time; they just leave it on the table. They all know I used to use drugs, so they never give me a lot more because it might be a trigger."

Sitting on the examining table, she picks up a pleat of her dress between two fingers and puts it down. Her situation in life requires a range of adjustments. She moves slowly, speaks slowly.

"I suppose they've given me more over the years, inflation you know, but they never really said and I never really thought about it. I probably make about six or seven hundred dollars a month. I never learned to be thrifty.

"If I needed $100, I can get it easily; I'd just call one of them. We're friends. We go out to dinner. I like to eat out and do common stuff like other people do. If they didn't pay me, I'd still benefit—nice gifts or trips. I know that sounds awful."

Once and Always

"I got SSDI [Social Security Disability Insurance] at eighteen for PTSD. Once disabled, always disabled, that's the way they've made it. I'm now thirty-five and want to work. I have Medicare and Medicaid. If I get off Medicare, I can't pay for my scripts and my visits."

"That wouldn't be good," I say. She's diligent about taking her anxiety medication.

"If I get a job without benefits, I could qualify for Obamacare, but that would take a while and I don't want to be uncovered. They can't simply move me from Medicare to Obamacare. To keep my medical coverage, I have to make less than $200 a week. I need a job with benefits or that pays enough so I can pay for benefits. But I can't get a job like that with my record."

One View of the Future

"I'm going down to the SSI office tomorrow to demand a trial," he says ruefully. "I want to file suit for wrongful death. If they make me go back to work and I die there, I want to hold SSI responsible."

Climate Change

"What's my job? Protect all wetlands. Conservation. I've been doing it for thirty years. The nature of the job is to fight with people."

He has a hard set to his mouth. I can tell he'd be difficult to argue with if he thought he was in the right.

"I regulate people's yards. The bad neighbor calls when he sees a pool going in next door and doesn't want his neighbor to be happy. He's just trying to get them in trouble. The pool person asks me, 'Why didn't they tell me I'd need to get a permit?'

"Early in my career most pools had to go. Not now. Some days I commit, but there are a lot of days when I just go home. When I turned fifty-nine I was out, the way I planned it. I'd collect 60 percent of my state salary and get another job. Then the governor changed and the retirement system changed. I got screwed. Now I don't think we need to protect all the wetland."

No Argument

"They kept my garage shut until I could produce some permits I'd never bothered to apply for, and it was just as well since I couldn't do heavy work for a few weeks while my wound healed."

He lifts his shirt to show me the scar on his left flank.

"To make up the lost cash, I did some landscaping and grass cutting. I trimmed the lawn of one of my regular customers. When I finished, the guy came outside to complain that he didn't need a cutting that day, even though the grass was six inches high. He wouldn't pay. He was trying to get over on me, but I didn't want to argue and get stabbed again.

"I could have put the guy who knifed me in jail, but I let it go with a ten-year no-contact order. I don't want that stabbing to rent space in my head."

UNDERGRADUATES

You have a 22 percent chance of not graduating from high school if you have lived in poverty, compared to 6 percent if you have never been poor. If you spent more than half your childhood in poverty, you're up to a 32 percent chance of dropping out.

Cakes: Perry

He seems lighter today, a boxer in the late rounds finding the energy to dance again.

"She bakes cakes and sells them in the neighborhood. Edith's her name. I just met her when I bought one of her cakes. Her son sold it to me, actually. He's twelve and looks like her, dark lashes.

"I asked him what he was going to do with the money.

"He said, 'Buy a sheep and raise him like a pet.'

"'In the apartment?' Edith asked. 'And who's paying for his food?'

Then to me, 'He won't usually talk to men.'

"She said I had a nice face, which isn't really true. The first time my mother saw me, newborn, her question was, 'Where'd he get that big nose?'

"I won't smile. That's how gross this boxer's mouth is to me."

Caffeinated

"I start at 6 A.M. at The Donut. I feel like I'm rushing as soon as I get there. Even though they've been open since five, the cream machine is empty, the ice machine is empty. My daughter comes with me. She plays on her Tablet until 7:30 and I walk her to school. Until she leaves, she talks to me, although I'm trying to take orders. She says, Mom, Mom, Mom. It's hard not to get mad at her or be mean to her—shhh, I keep saying, or I can't do my job and I won't get paid."

I can feel her tension—work pulling her one way, her daughter pulling another. Her eczema is acting up; she has a rash on her hands.

"With the headset on, I don't have to talk to the customers at the counter. I write down what the drivers say into the microphone. I do the coffee, not the food. I write down the orders so no one around has to ask. People who work with me walk like snails and I'm frantic. There's no rush, but for me there is. They call me Huff and Puff, as in blow your house down, because I'm always aggravated. I can't get it all done. My brain is everywhere. But I have to pull it all together for the five cars in the drive thru."

Office Politics

"I'm fine one minute, then I explode. I vent for ten minutes and I'm fine. Sometimes I have to walk out of the building. I puke before I go to work. I'm there until eight every night. I never take a vacation. I don't get help. I can't take it anymore. I do everything and don't get recognized. They bypassed me when filling the manager position. You think it's because I have a bad attitude?"

He gives a nervous little laugh, and again refuses medication for his heartburn.

Proof

"The last eight years I worked, I was paid under the table. But the company played me dirty. I can't prove I worked for them. I should get $1,000 a month from unemployment now, but I'm getting like $800 and I can't do anything about it unless I bring them pay stubs and I never had pay stubs."

Putting on a Show

"I work with disabled adults. It's like a day care. At work, there's lots of being 'on,' like a clown. I constantly have to act happy. I take them to the mall or bowling.

"I get this call from work last week. 'There's a situation going on and you may be somewhat involved,' my supervisor says. 'What situation?' I ask. She wouldn't tell me details, but she said they would need me *not* to come in until they finish the investigation. 'Don't come in. I'll be in touch,' my supervisor says.

"I'm on administrative leave. After five days I call back because they still haven't called or given me my schedule for the next week. 'We're not finished. Maybe next week.'

"My daughter's disabled, but not as severe as my clients. My child has to get the best of me, but I come home exhausted. I'm a single parent; I do everything on my own.

"I can't go another week without income."

When she cries, she takes great heaving breaths. I hand her a box of tissues. I have the dreadful conviction that her life is as luckless as mine is fortunate.

"Before I felt underwater, but I could come up for air. Now I come up for air, but I can't breathe because I'm already sinking again."

Nostalgia

"Man, what I did to get the money to get the drugs. The drive I had. I'd make money out of nothing. I wasn't afraid to work. I always found something. After a storm, I'd do tree work, cleaning people's yards. I'd go door to door looking for work. I had no insurance for climbing the trees—I had to lie about that if they asked—but I knew how to keep a job."

Hard Bargain

"I used to own a laundromat. I bought it with a small business loan and money I saved. Sixty machines. My wife and I worked it for three years. There was no money being made."

I like his shift into the passive tense, the impersonal note of destiny. I can see where this is headed.

"The landlord wanted to raise the rent on the place and I told him, 'If you raise the rent, I'll move out and people around here will smash every window and you'll never rent the place again. You need to lower the rent.'"

He rubs his face and rearranges himself in his chair, pleased to have done what needed to be done, and to have surprised me a little.

Savers

"I started a new job at Savers, shipping and receiving—people drop stuff off and we go through it to see what we can sell—and I'm trying to fit in. I randomly say something stupid. I ask questions I already know the answers to, like, 'How am I doing?' I just say shit that comes into my head."

My mind wanders as his does. I wonder where he's now living—still with his mother? I'll ask.

"I'm with one of the managers going through things and I pick up a pair of old Reeboks and I ask him, 'Remember these?' I'm talking about how out of style they are. He looks at me funny. He calls me into his office later and says, 'We're having a problem with you. You can't take anything home.' 'I didn't,' I say. 'I didn't steal nothing.' He says, 'Remember those shoes you liked? You shouldn't take them home.' 'I'd never take anything. That's stealing,' I say."

A Mother's Eye

"I lost the job, but I got a new job making $11 an hour at the Dollar Store. I just got promoted to manager. My friend calls and says, 'You want to detail a few cars?' I know I can make $200 in a day, so I can't afford to pass on it. I call in sick despite the promotion."

He wears his baseball cap backward. His optimism is unstoppable. I appreciate his desire to make things better.

"My friend does the shampoo and wet vac. I do the glaze and wax. Then we bring the car by my mother's house for her to have a look at what we might have missed. She has an eye for it. She used to own a car wash. She usually catches me on the door jambs and the rear-view mirror. We give her a cut."

Degrees

"I went over to the community college to sign up to learn how to use this expensive machine, a 3D printer. Starting next summer, if I can get financial aid. I don't know why I went, really. I'm more of a certificate kind of guy than a college guy. I'm thinking of doing a CDL, certified [commercial] driver's license. That's a six-week class rather than four years. I won't have any loans to pay off. You get a diploma after either one."

Accidents Happen

"I was working in this warehouse with a forklift, and I put the fork through the metal ceiling. The pile of clothes was too high, and I was trying to put this bale on top. I call outside to this guy working with me who started the same day I did: 'Dude, bring the duct tape.'

"All they did to prepare me was have me watch a video, and then they put me on the thing. What did they expect? No one's perfect. I'm not telling anyone. If they find out, I'll deal with it. They'll probably dock my pay."

"Shouldn't they?" I ask.

Dessert: Perry

"I asked Edith out to dinner."

He took a large breath, held it in his overinflated lungs while his cheeks puffed out. He expelled the air slowly through his nostrils.

"Good for you," I say. "It sounded at the last visit like you were headed in that direction." I wonder if she has opinions about his mismatched clothes.

"She cleans offices and sells the cakes to supplement. She makes $16,000 a year, not bad for a family of two, since she spends zero on groceries with her food stamps and what she gets from pantries, and she lives subsidized, right here in my building. She has $800 in savings. She told me about her savings during the salad course. She puts away twenty bucks a month. She's smart with money.

"She even had her legal fees paid for after her ex hit her. He made good money, but he kept it to himself, Edith said.

"She let me pay for dinner. I bought a brownie for Joseph. For his sheep."

I could tell he felt triumphant, and that made me happy.

Speak Softly and Carry

"I'm working extra shifts at Wendy's, 4 P.M. to 2 A.M. six days a week. Me and another girl close the place. I walk home at 3 A.M. I don't want a car—insurance, payments, gas. I'd rather walk. I have a big knife."

I nod, silently accepting her acceptance of a violent world. Despite the real risk, she seems secure.

The Arts

"Work's all around me. Auto detailing, yard service. You just have to have the nerve to go up to people."

He has an innocence; he doesn't take personally what the world throws at him.

"But the only thing I actually enjoy is music. I got a couple of turntables, an MPC [music production center]. I'm doing samples, splits. Been doing it nine years, since I was seventeen. There's no future in it for me. I'd like to do commercials, or the music at the end of *Law and Order*. But I'll never get that. What it comes down to is laziness. My girlfriend's supporting me right now. I know how to make money, that's not the problem. I'd just rather work with music even if I never get paid."

Growth

"We grow medical marijuana for the state and make about $1,000 a month, but $200 goes to electric for grow lights. I never touch the stuff. I could care less. I'm on to bigger things: heroin."

Meat Market

"My brother and I were partners. He was cheap. He used an 8-cent roll for our veal parm sandwiches because he was buying lousy stuff from a friend rather than spending on better rolls. He had me selling frozen turkey as if it was fresh to get 70 cents more a pound. He forced me to lie. People would call the store: 'If this is fresh, why is there ice in the bird?'

"But then he starts letting his wife use the company credit card for tennis lessons. This was the man who judged me day to day. My brother is not an idiot, just a barbarian, good at talking bullshit. But he had to make a choice: me or his wife. The last time I talked to him was 2010."

Grandparent Program

"Age sixty-one, I quit as a respiratory tech after fifteen years because of herniated disks. I took my $879 a month and moved into section 8. Rent's $254; $168 for my TV and phone bundle; $40 a month paying off my bedroom set, and $100 a month on food. I don't eat much, mostly bagels and frozen fish, and I like broccoli. I have no savings in a bank. I do have a special something set aside though; they'll never know what."

"No one needs to know," I say.

"I did try to go back to work in a grandparent program for disadvantaged kids. But they were disrespectful. They cursed; they were mean. They had problems, I knew; they were on medication; some had been abused since age six. But I didn't like hollering like the other aides. I didn't want to discipline other people's children all day, no matter what I was paid."

Return of Religion

"I'm working really hard at $9 an hour, but $360 at the end of the week doesn't really cut it. Maybe I'll start going to church again."

Blue Chip

"I breed bullies—half pit bull, half bulldog. You can make your own mutants. I jerk them off and sell the semen for $2,500. The crazier they look, the more people want to spend. The dog only has to see the bag now and he gets off, as long as there's a female in the room. My favorite is called Dow Jones—she makes me money."

Bookkeeping

She always has a coffee with her, which she raises to her lip-sticked mouth.

"Although I used to be a bookkeeper, I'm on SSDI and not supposed to be working. I work twenty-five hours a week under the table. If anyone knew I had a job, I'd have to give up my insurance, and then I'd never be able to pay for my meds, and if I didn't take my meds I wouldn't be able to go to work.

"I pick up the rent from the addicts at a halfway house. I have them leave the money in a lockbox so they don't know who picks it up. I wouldn't want someone to rat on me so I'd lose my SSDI. I know someone would; I was an addict once."

Tough: Perry

"Edith doesn't really have friends in the building either."

He's a little sad, a little pleased.

"She tells me people here are lazy. She shows me shoes she bought twenty years ago where she just had the bottoms replaced for $3. 'I use them, but would anyone else around here do that?' she asks me. She has no patience for her neighbors. I used to box, but she's tougher on people than I am."

THREE MEN

The combined wealth of Bill Gates,

Jeff Bezos, and Warren Buffett is equal

to the wealth of half of the entire U.S.

population.

SELF

TO DIE FOR

Children aged nine to sixteen years old living below the poverty line are three times likelier to admit to wanting to die than children who aren't, after taking into account symptoms of anxiety or depression, alcohol use, and drug use.

Nails: Perry

"Edith tells me proudly she's never been on welfare. She's always worked, even if she took food stamps. She pointed out this woman in the building who makes her hair blond and has fake nails. To keep her nails good, she has to go every week to a nail shop, Edith tells me, disgusted. 'Thirty dollars a visit. The money they take out of *my* pay goes to her for *that?*'"

I can see how Perry is falling for her, and it makes me think about how he will be transformed.

Perspective

"Poor? No. I live in the United States and I have running water and a bathroom. It's nice to get new things, but phones and cars don't mean anything. I have what I need to live. As a kid, we didn't have a drier. My clothes were wet when I went to school. That was the only time I ever felt poor."

Between Two Men

"My son's moving out. My husband's a jerk. Last night I had to stand in the way so the two of them didn't fight. They just don't get along, and never did. Last night they were arguing because when my son gets money, he gives his father ten bucks or a sack of weed. But when his father gets money, he doesn't give nothing to my son. My son says, 'I pay half the rent here and he can't give me a lousy ten bucks?' He was so angry he knocked all my knickknacks all over the place in the living room, my ceramic bears, my glass cups."

She seems outraged, but I can't tell by which part. I know she's stood between these two men before.

"He didn't touch the baby pictures, luckily. I screamed, 'If you don't cut it out, I'll call the cops.' I thought I'd have an asthma attack. Maybe if he moves out, my husband and me will get along better. Guess what, we won't."

Irony

"I spend $20 a month on a cremation policy I started thirteen years ago. It was going for $5,000. That's what you do when you're in the Fire Department."

The Cost of Addiction

"I'm an addict in every sense. With my last three bucks I bought Nutella, and it was gone the same day. I used one spoon, and whipped cream. My dog likes whipped cream, and he followed me into the kitchen every time for leftovers, but I could see he had this look in his eye: you really ought to stop."

Three Questions

"I need to think of myself as poor again. Doing that, I once saved $5,000. I could buy porterhouse steaks then," she says. "My rule used to be: lock up $100 a month. I used to have two credit cards. But just because I had them didn't mean I needed to use them. When I had money, I bought DVDs and clothes. Now I go into a store with three questions: do you need it, do you want it, can you live without it?"

She has hopes, but they are infused with a realistic awareness.

Plans

"Food and housing aren't a problem, I just don't do other stuff."

Sometimes when a patient starts to say something I know will be painful, I look down rather than directly at them.

"My phone's broken, that would cost $100. I need a haircut, and my son does too. Can't do that. When I went to community college, I got bus passes, but I don't go anymore, so I lost my bus rides," he says. "The most in savings I ever had was $600. I'd like a car, but I have to save. I also owe $350 just to get my license back. Then I'd have to up my game to be able to pay for car insurance."

Who's the Winner?

"My wife takes the car in to get fixed. It comes home with a noise. She takes it back and they say they don't know what the noise is. They're trying to gouge us, I know. They say, maybe it's the spark plugs; we can replace them. That's $400. My wife says no and brings the car home again with the noise. I call them and scream, 'How can you run a business that way?' I say to my wife, 'Why didn't you leave the car and tell them to figure it out and fix the noise?' She won't fight with them. Now she's fighting with me. She says, 'I can't win with you either.'"

Cashing Out

"My father died when I was twenty," he says.

His chair scrapes the linoleum floor, and one leg leaves a black line.

"I was sitting in this restaurant and I got a feeling. Something comes over me that says, 'Go home.' I walk in the door and the phone rings. It's the hospital. They say to come right over. He was already dead. He had his shirt ripped open; he was still warm when I kissed him. He had a Quinella ticket in his pocket, a winning ticket. He went out a winner. I went back to the casino a few weeks later and picked up the cash."

Custody

"After my heart attack I quit working because of ill health, and I don't even have the gas money to see my eight-year-old son who lives with my ex an hour away. I try to get to him once a month like it says in our custody agreement. But I can't even do that. Try telling an eight-year-old you can't see him because you don't have the money."

Sometimes what I hear is so unbearably sad I have to leave the room.

Allowance

"I'm sixty-four and I don't know if I'll ever be clean. Using is just part of my makeup. Once I start with that feeling, I give up. Even if I went away for thirty days I still have to go home. They say the more time sober, the better, but I've never had thirty days my whole life. I get depressed about that sometimes. Why can't I be normal? What would my father, a hard-working man, say?"

"What do you *think* he would say?" I ask. I haven't heard much about his father. Did he drink every day also? We're both distracted by the ambulance noise outside the window.

"My wife says she has three kids, me and the other two. She leaves in the morning and gives me four bucks. What am I gonna do with four bucks? She takes my keys with her too, and at night, so I don't go out. I get an $800 pension from the union every month. All that and my wife gives me only $4 so I have to borrow money for breakfast."

Interest: Perry

"Here's the amazing thing to me about Edith: she takes her son on vacation. He's twelve and he's been out of the country twice: Puerto Rico and the Dominican Republic. Since I left the service I haven't been on a plane. But she's figured out a way to take Joseph."

He is pleased by this thought. He struggles to communicate well. He has islands of sweat under his arms.

"She finds these credit cards that are interest free for a year. She signs up, uses it to take a trip, pays it off from her savings, and closes the card. She says she's never paid interest."

Left Behind

"My friend died and he left me $30,000 and $92,000 more in an IRA. One of his sisters called and told me. 'John left you his work policy,' she said, and gave me this number to call. When I went in to sign the papers at his union office (he used to install HVACs) the lady there told me John's brothers and sisters had been calling asking wasn't there some mistake; they didn't understand why he gave me the money. The union mailed me the two checks two weeks later," she says.

Her eyes are rimmed in red.

"I had to do the right thing, so I paid for the funeral. The rest I signed over to my mother so my food stamps people or whoever couldn't get at the money he'd left me.

"But I don't do well with my mother. We argue. I have a personality like my dad, not like my mother. He died when I was sixteen. I'm that kind of person who goes in not knowing anyone and leaves knowing everyone. I look like my dad. Like him, I swear every other word. But she's my mother, and for a woman there's no worse pain than having a child, so I owe her."

Anniversaries

"Sometimes I can't breathe good. I feel uneasy. And if I drink it calms it down. My last drink was yesterday. Vodka, $2 for a half pint. Chernobyl water. That's half the four bucks my wife gives me for breakfast. Today I went to two meetings, the first at 7 A.M. Breakfast at Bill's, I call it. I tell 'em I'm celebrating one day sober. They handed me the Big Book to read. A guy comes up to me afterward and asks me to talk on an audiobook for kids he's making. I guess because my voice goes up and down like kids like. Imagine. Me, reading to kids."

He has the expression of someone who's said something extraordinary. "I can definitely imagine that," I say.

"I belong in a nut house, but I could make a few bucks reading. It's our fortieth wedding anniversary coming up. If I earn the cash, I'll take her out for dinner for sticking around. I'm sure she'll order veal parm, penne too, probably."

Checkup

"I've been bad," she says. "I want to get checked. Bad, you know what I'm saying, right? Bad. I want to be sure I'm good. Clean when I go back to him. What does it cost to get the test?"

Less than Zero

"My son works. He's twenty-seven and he makes more than I do. He still comes over to borrow $20 and doesn't pay me back. He says he's out of cash. Why's he broke? I wonder. I used to think he spent it on porn. Now I think he goes to the track like my father did. I don't ask. What's he going to say, 'Dad, I lose money all the time'? At least he don't drink."

What Money Could Buy

"I've never been with a woman. The first vagina I saw was on a movie screen when I was twenty-one. I live a deformed life as a woman. When men look at me, are attracted to me, it's not because I was a man. I am not comfortable in a room of women or of straight people. I'm sixty-three. I was this way since I was nineteen. You gotta put in your time. Caitlyn Jenner, that's not right at sixty. If I could have made love to a woman and had children, I wouldn't have gone this route. How can you feel feminine doing masculine things like making love to a woman?"

She has large hands and a small nose; different parts of her don't go together. She comes in every few months for her hormone prescription.

"I don't think of myself as transgender. I have a deformity. I was just born with a penis, a deformity. There are lots of men who like to wear women's clothes. I'm not attracted to gay men. I would never say I'm gay. The straight men I'm with meet me as a woman and later on I tell them, 'I'm a woman with a deformity and I can't afford the surgery.'"

Poetry

"My mother's always been a heavy drinker. When she decided to quit (I was nine months pregnant at the time), she went out the door saying, 'Tonight will be my last hurrah!' On the way home from the bar she hit a fifteen-year-old girl who was walking. Luckily she didn't kill her. I got a call from the police, 'Will you come bail your mother out?' I called her husband, my stepfather, and asked him why he hadn't been called. They'd been fighting that night, he said. 'Screw her. I'm not bailing her.' So they called me. When I spoke to her, all she said was, 'I've been cuffed and stuffed and my man won't pay enough.' Like she'd been writing that poem all night."

On the Way Out

"My father's in the ICU on his way out, and I only wish I could push him quicker. I want his houses and his car, a Chevrolet. When I was a baby he left my mother with a box of baking soda in the refrigerator. Meanwhile he was giving $100 tips to some waitress."

He speaks with distaste, as if he's about to spit.

"If my mother was a guy, she would have been the head of organized crime. The gangsters in our neighborhood would kill people and confess to her. My father was only half a gangster. That's a gangster who never made a dime so he had to go to work."

Thinking Things

"I think about what I have to do and don't get nothing done. I think so many things I don't do the one thing I need to do. I overthink everything. If I don't buy an Adderall, I don't think I'll finish anything."

Monopoly

"I pimped out my girlfriend. I filmed her with a judge, a married man, and now he knows I can extort him. I don't want cash. I'd rather have a Get Out of Jail Free card."

I wonder what his mother the gangster would say.

Love: Perry

"She has her own washing machine. Her son has his own room. But most importantly, Edith has ACs in all the rooms of her apartment like I do."

I remember him telling me, months before, that the building charges him $11 per month per AC. There is a new softness to the hard lines of his face. His eyes are like dark stones at the bottom of a stream.

"I think I'm in love."

Sympathy

"My brother called me from the hospital two days after they locked him up. He'd done it at home and wandered bleeding out onto the street. When he called, he said, 'My wrists really hurt.' 'What did you expect?' I asked. 'Can you buy me gloves?' he asked."

Mixed Emotions

"I'm managing this building where students live. I go in to fix the sink. On the table of the living room is a bottle of cocaine and a spoon," she says. "Who leaves that out, knowing workers are coming over? I call my buddy who's there with me to come take a look, and he says, 'Walk away.'"

"Usually a good idea," I say.

"I wouldn't have thought about it twice if it weren't for my mother. I needed something to get out of my head. I usually do the right thing. But last night, my mother called me at 8 P.M. She said, 'Vera's over, we're eating dinner.' She's slurring her words. We'd already talked at four that afternoon as we do every day. I said, 'Ma, you're drinking. Stop drinking.' 'Okay,' she said, 'but if I don't, you'll never know.'

"This morning Vera called me, 'We're at the hospital. Your mother fell and broke her wrist.' I should have gone over last night, but I was at the casino, losing."

Sophie's Choice

"This guy owes me 200 bucks. He's late with his payment, and he knows I can't let him be late. I take out a knife. I see he's afraid. I hand it to him, and I say, 'If you cut me, add $100. If I have to cut myself, I'm adding $200.'"

Training

"My Get Out of Jail Free card didn't work."

I had been wondering why he'd missed his last appointment.

"When I was in, I had a good job; eighty cents a day into my fund. I was training dogs for handicapped people, like people in wheelchairs. I was always good with animals. The dogs are the ones that don't quite make it as Guiding Eye dogs. These are the dogs that are a little less confident, or a little more fearful. But they can still turn on lights, open the refrigerator, let a person know that a phone was ringing or there was someone at the door. I always identified with those dogs, although I had a worse temper."

Alone Time

"If I have extra money, I buy me a couple of beers. If I ever had $60, I'd go out on a fishing boat. If I had lots of money, I'd buy a yacht to fish from myself. If I was rich, I'd buy my wife a house next to mine."

Don't Touch

"The asshole in my house, my daughter's father, stays with her when I work at night."

I slide my chair away from her a few inches to give her room. She's come back to see me after a few missed appointments.

"Yesterday he went in my wallet and took $20. When I found out, I needed to take a step back before I put him through the wall. If I hit him, I'll lose my daughter. She don't talk so she just looked at me. She won't come to me when I'm angry. She can feel it."

Worlds

"You can't ask my daughter. She doesn't talk. But she watches. If I start smoking again, she watches me. She sees me cry every day.

"When she comes home from school at 11:20, for the next eight hours I can't wash dishes, talk on the phone, use the bathroom. I have to do everything for her. I don't know what she wants, but it's never enough. I can't get mad at her. She's my world."

She finally asks me to help her find family services, someone to give her advice about her daughter. I feel afraid for her, a sensation like when I'm swimming in the bay and I suddenly feel I'm alone, and I swim hard toward land.

"I have repetition in my life, but no stability. I'm still waiting for the good days that are coming. I'm existing, but I feel dead. At best, we sit on couch and I get on my phone to answer surveys for money.

"I rant and rave. When I'm ready to pop off, I meditate; I put the ocean on my phone. Should I walk away?"

It wouldn't seem like an incomprehensible crime, I think.

"Everyone has walked away from me. She needs me, and that's what holds me back. But if I do, my son Jesse has money for her in the safe."

Blessings

"I get $764 a month. I give $12.50 to my church. More if I can. It all comes around, though. I told my minister that my sister died and I couldn't pay for the ticket to Baltimore, and he paid for me, by train even. And he bought me a Bible with large print to take with me."

Prices: Perry

"When Edith invites me for dinner, I bring a bottle of wine. It cost me $14.99. At the meal, she asks me why I don't drink. I tell her the story.

"My father sat me down when I was ten and filled up two shot glasses.

'Drink it,' he said.

'I don't want to.'

He hit me.

'Drink it,' he said.

So I drank it.

He hit me again.

'You drank that like a pro. You've been drinking before.'

'I haven't. I've been watching you.'

I hadn't bought a bottle of wine for anyone, including myself, in twenty years."

"You're a new man," I say.

"Prices have gone up."

Have Strive

"I did three and half for cocaine possession, the last year in minimum, working in a restaurant. I got paid, but I didn't care about the money. I sent it all to my wife and child. They had to feed me in jail anyway. Now that I'm back, I'm a go-getter. I breed my bullies."

With exacting fingers he smooths out the creases of the paper bag he's carrying.

"You just have to live every day like you're hungry. You chase it. If you don't make it, you can't feed your kids, and I will *always* feed my kids. You got to have strive."

One Question

"How would I like my life to be better? If I was downtown and saw a SALE sign, I'd go in instead of thinking, 'I hope it's there next time when I have money with me.'"

Wants

"Before I went to jail, I always found ways to get things. I never understood the word 'want.' If I wanted clothes or sneakers, I'd steal them or I'd sell drugs to buy them. Now, if I'm lucky, I do demo work for $800 a month. It gets the aggression out. I'm knocking down walls and also saving for this motorcycle I want."

Who's the Idiot?

"I let an idiot in my house, someone I've known since I was a kid. I went outside to smoke. She was in the house looking after my daughter, I thought."

Arms implacably folded, she's shaking her head.

"That afternoon I go to take my pain medication, and half the pills are gone. I think maybe I misplaced them. I'm absentminded. Then I start screaming at my boyfriend. But he wasn't even around in the morning; he didn't take the pills. I can't call the cops, they wouldn't believe me.

"I can't afford to pay cash for a refill, and my insurance won't let me get more early. Now who's the idiot?"

Caught between
Two Women

His hands are clenched in his lap.

"My daughter was managing my mom's money while living with her. My daughter had cancer and a morphine pump, and after they took the pump out she started using pills, and that's when she stole from my mother. She stopped paying the mortgage, and my eighty-six-year-old mother lost her home and claimed bankruptcy.

"My daughter went to jail for three weeks, and someone decided they didn't have enough evidence to sentence her for longer. Now I have to choose between my mother and my daughter, who will be part of my life. My mother has a restraining order on my daughter. I'd like to ask my daughter why she did it, but if I talk to her, I know she'll tell my mother."

Big Brother

"The whole American government is a monster. Brilliant people who know who buys what."

I haven't seen him in a long time. I wonder if he's been hospitalized for the voices he hears. He sees the world as adversarial, and despite his history, that seems reasonable to me.

"Around here, the politicians keep screwing up. The city buys buses that don't work, so the fares go up.

"One of the few luxuries of the poor is cigarettes, but they keep taxing them. They want to take our cigarettes away. I see them looking out of those bank windows downtown thinking, 'They have no money, but they have money to smoke?' They blame the poor for being poor."

Looking Back

"I was going home from the grocery store this morning, thinking about what I'll do when I wake up tomorrow morning with no job to go to now that I'm laid off. When I reached my corner, this man stood rattling the coins in his red plastic cup, his arm outstretched. He was wearing a black T-shirt. He tried to catch my eye. I walked by without putting anything in.

"When I was two steps past, he said, 'Should have.'"

CHILD'S DECISION

Eat the school lunch at school, or save it for the weekend.

Concluding Thoughts

America is money. That's how America got to be America, and that's what America is and will always be. America is an invoice.

Patients pay to see me. The only money that changes hands is at the front desk, where the secretary asks for payment for the visit. The secretary makes demands, touches the cash, lets them in. I never touch their money.

It gets tricky if she tries to help by not asking for a co-payment: the insurers would hold us in breach of contract. They want every patient who sees a doctor to have skin in the game — if the insurer has to pay, the patient does too.

A few times over the years I've bought from them clams or a hat or candles or hand-knitted socks so they would have a few more dollars in their pocket that day. I've taken out my wallet and we've traded. They name the price. Honor and a good name, that's how to do business.

The gospel of having money, that's what everything gets reduced to. That's what everyone is fighting for. No one can be trusted when it comes to money. "I'm not a rich doctor like you," more than one patient has said to me. It's true: I never had to fight for money. I give advice from within my life of greater security. Can I possibly get it right, in their best interests?

Can I feel what they feel? Things break all the time — the car, the TV, the AC, a beer bottle, a lightbulb. Can I feel them breaking? Their lives are about fixing or getting down on one knee and picking up the pieces. People break. Fingers. Noses. Fevers. Hearts.

Broken sleep. They can't sleep. They're all tired. What keeps them up at night? Dreams? They're all worried about kids, but what scares them, what makes them feel hunted? What's buried beneath?

Money, always money. What they owe. The down payment, the rent. The bad deal they still need to pay off. The perpetual price of living. You can have it if you can afford it; can't if you can't. You start with nothing and the IRS takes *that* away. You know the story. The symptoms of the American Dream. They're sick of it.

So they come to see me.

Often when my patients talk about money it is unprompted, spontaneous, inserted into a story they're telling. I ask for the details. I have come to think of these conversations about money with patients — which certainly don't occur at every visit, but only when pertinent, and only with patients I've come to know — as a form of preventive care.

Feeling a bit more in control of their finances, or less out of control, allows patients the mental space to perhaps make clearer decisions, health decisions included. So when the decision to pay off a credit card bill comes along, and they share their thinking (and the bill itself) with me, it not only gives me insight into that patient's home life but also allows me a chance to give advice.

Preventive care is sometimes more important than the physical exam at a given appointment, and so my visits don't typically run long—I don't like to keep other patients waiting. Listening is of course central to all primary care medicine, and every physician has to hear what's important to patients beyond the chief complaint, which is sometimes only a small part of the reason a patient came in.

What does this mean for the role of the clinician? Clinicians remain responsible for fixing the immediate problem but must, we believe, eventually also grapple with the underlying concerns. The issues of inadequate housing, inadequate food, limited access to addiction treatment, and terrible neighborhoods *are* medical problems. But these issues are larger than any individual clinician caring for an individual patient. Clinicians can choose to be advocates, voices for health outside of the hospital or clinic, or they can advocate that their hospital or clinic embrace these issues with fervor.

Listening to the stories of the poor led me to change my career. I moved from this primary care practice to a new position as the leader of a health policy department at a public health school. But there is something unique and irreplaceable about each individual that cannot be seen in data collected from across an entire population. I hope that the stories I've written here, that have changed my life, will inspire and move others to address the issues of poverty in America.

A COVID Afterword

"The guys who drive during the day get hazard pay, time and a half," my patient says, annoyed. He'd been working third shift in a liquor warehouse for just under a year. He'd wanted to be a driver but had failed the written part of the test three times. "They don't even restock the shelves anymore. They just drop the full pallet in front of the liquor store and drive off." It's April and my patients and I are two months into full-time talk of the pandemic. "Like COVID is around only when it's light outside," he adds sarcastically. During our telemedicine visit, he can see me sitting on the white couch in my den with a blank wall behind me—a neutral background so he gets no sense of my life, my economics—and I can see him sitting in his cluttered living room with its tower of CDs and a Led Zeppelin poster. "We got more risk of infection at night loading the trucks, seven of us in that warehouse. With the heavy lifting it's hard to breathe with a face mask."

As a doctor, I am in one of the few professions where we already wear masks (along with nail salon workers, carpenters, and hazmat material removers). Now we all wear them. In the first eight weeks of the shut down, 30 million Americans lost their jobs. My medical office is closed, but I'm still employed. Safe even, working from home and conferring with patients through my practice's computer network, wearing the same button-down shirts I would wear in my office, but in jeans, which they cannot see. There are no physical exams anymore, but there is more time to talk. The telehealth camera lets me into my patients' apartments filled with children's toys, piles of laundry, the sounds of dishes getting washed, giant TV screens, and Styrofoam take-out boxes. At home, they seem more relaxed, clumsier, more forgetful and fun, emotionally sturdier in a way, inviting me into their lives. At times I feel a little guilty, studying them in this new way, as if I'm outside, staring in through their windows.

The ones who have kept their jobs are grateful. One with a sense of humor about his career in waste management says, laughing, "The garbage never stops." His work, so embedded in reality, remains the source of a paycheck. Another patient is taking a break from looking for a job. "What's the point right now?" he asks. "No one's working anyway." He, like other patients I visit with through my laptop screen, is cutting back on his spending for now, skipping meals, waiting for his government stimulus check to arrive. I ask several of them what they will use the anticipated twelve hundred dollars for. One says, "Rainy day fund." Another says, "Cigarettes and snacks." Another says, "New brake pads." A fourth says, "I won't get the money. The feds will keep it for the child support I owe."

As always, I listen for the eerie minor key of despair in their voices. Locked in, they trade old problems for new ones: More time with the mother whose memory is gone. More time with the teenage son's older boyfriend who seems to have moved in and has no money to contribute to the food or rent. There is plenty of emotion and restlessness. Almost always, someone else is in the room when we're talking, just beyond the screen. Sometimes my patients turn the camera so I can meet this person with whom they share real-world problems and misunderstandings and reconciliations.

My patients want me to know more, now that I'm in their homes. They want me to see what they have to put up with. No one rushes away as they did when visiting my office, telling me they have to get back to work or pick up a child at school. I am moved when one jokingly offers to make me coffee. "What do you think of my place?" some ask expectantly. In the old days they asked, "How do my lungs sound?" We are connected in new ways through these house calls. I can feel the enclosed repetition of all of our lives, and how it protects us.

They know it wasn't anyone's fault, this pause in the world. The virus has brought a period of uncertainty that will stretch into months. They are waiting for the next check, the next break. They will have to decide what to keep, what to forgo. I will try to help. Each one asks when our next visit will be. They all tell me to be safe, be well.

CPSIA information can be obtained
at www.ICGtesting.com
Printed in the USA
LVHW071714211120
672337LV00013B/234